Sarah Flower, a leading nutritionist and author of many cookery books, is passionate about healthy eating and a keen advocate of the sugar-free and low-carb way of eating. She has trained with The Real Meal Revolution, originally set up by Professor Noakes and Jonno Proudfoot, both of whom advise banting/LCHF (low carbohydrate, high fat) and is now herself a banting coach in the UK.

Sarah writes for a number of publications, including the *Daily Mail*, *Top Santé* magazine and *Healthista*. She appears regularly on BBC Radio Devon.

Also by Sarah Flower

The Busy Mum's Plan-ahead Cookbook
The Sugar-Free Family Cookbook
Eat Well, Spend Less
The Healthy Lifestyle Diet Cookbook
The Healthy Halogen Cookbook
The Healthy Slow Cooker Cookbook
Perfect Baking with Your Halogen Oven
Halogen Cooking for Two
The Everyday Halogen Family Cookbook
The Everyday Halogen Oven Cookbook
Slow Cook, Fast Food
The Low-Carb Slow Cooker

Eating to Beat Type 2 Diabetes

The low-carb way to reverse insulin resistance and control diabetes

Sarah Flower

A How To Book

ROBINSON

ROBINSON

First published in Great Britain in 2018 by
Robinson

A CIP catalogue record for this book
is available from the British Library.

ISBN: 978-1-47214-117-0

Typeset by Basement Press, Glaisdale
Printed and bound in Great Britain by CPI Group
(UK) Ltd, Croydon, CR0 4YY

Papers used by Robinson are
from well-managed forests and other
sustainable sources.

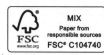

MIX
Paper from
responsible sources
FSC® C104740

Robinson
An imprint of
Little, Brown Book Group
Carmelite House
50 Victoria Embankment
London EC4Y 0DZ

An Hachette UK Company
www.hachette.co.uk

www.littlebrown.co.uk

The recommendations in this book are solely
intended as education and information and
should not be taken as medical advice.

How To Books are published by Robinson, an
imprint of Little, Brown Book Group. We
welcome proposals from authors who have
first-hand experience of their subjects.
Please set out the aims of your book, its
target market and its suggested contents in
an email to howtobooks@littlebrown.co.uk

Thank you to all my clients who have put their trust in me and are now on the road to better health. All my love to my very patient husband for putting up with my obsession with work and having to taste all my experimental recipes.

Contents

INTRODUCTION

I don't think I have ever been as passionate about a way of eating as I am with low carb. The results have been mind-blowing. Just changing my diet to eating real food, limiting carbohydrates and sugar, and avoiding grains appears to have a dramatic, positive effect on health. This is not a fad diet. It is not depriving; it is giving you your life back.

I have been low carb, sugar free for a few years now. My health started to deteriorate as I approached forty. Typical 'fat, female and forty' I believe is the terminology. This was totally the opposite of what should have happened. I was vegetarian from my teens. As a nutritionist, I practised what I preached and ate a diet rich in whole grains, vegetables, fruit and smoothies. I didn't eat junk food or processed food, yet the weight started to pile on, and I felt sluggish and under par. I also developed fatty liver – not the best advert for a nutritionist!

Switching to low carb has been life-changing: my energy has returned, my weight has dropped and I feel so much better. The more I researched this diet, the more empowered I became. Friends and family soon followed suit. My nutritional clients who suffered from IBS, migraines, arthritis and high blood pressure reported amazing positive changes in their health, with blood sugars normalising. Could eliminating most carbohydrates from your diet really reverse some of the most crippling diseases? There is some amazing research going on using the LCHF (low-carb healthy-fat) diet to fight cancer, prevent Alzheimer's, and most exciting of all is to see remission of Type 2 diabetes. We must call this 'remission' rather than 'reversal'. Remission warns you that you will always have to watch your carbohydrate and sugar intake. If you started to eat high carbs and sugars again, you would see a return of Type 2 diabetes, so this must be a lifestyle change rather than a short-term diet.

One of my clients (let's call her Jenny) was in a bad way. Jenny was a difficult case: she lived alone in a bedsit, was T2 diabetic, had high blood pressure, was morbidly obese and was house-bound due to mobility and mental-health problems. She had no energy, felt physically ill and had very low mood. She had pretty much given up.

When she first started on the low-carb diet, she felt nervous but excited and motivated. She couldn't get her head around the fact that this diet was suitable for T2 diabetics. Doctors, nurses and dieticians all advised her to eat carbs, so reversing that thinking wasn't easy. Even now, having demonstrated success, she is still being told by her diabetic nurse and GP to be careful eating fats, while carbohydrates and sugars are not even mentioned.

Jenny decided to follow the Diet Doctor weekly menu plans (www.dietdoctor.com). She was not a keen cook, so this worked brilliantly for her. She could order all the ingredients online and found the recipes easy to follow.

Prior to following this way of eating, Jenny's blood-glucose levels were consistently in the high teens. Within a week they were down to the mid-teens, and six months later they were down to 7. Her HbA1C was over 100 in January. By March, a few weeks after starting this way of eating it was down to 87, in April 66, and in June 57. Her cholesterol went from 5.5 to 4.5. Best of all, she has lost weight, has more energy and is going out.

Lifestyle changes can be hard to implement, but try to focus on the positives. You really don't have to go without when you follow this way of eating. I have tried to include many family-favourite recipes so that you don't feel you are missing out. Remember to empower yourself with information, and please use the references at the back of this book. Additionally, there are some amazing websites, YouTube videos and leading experts to follow. T2 diabetes can take 10 years off your life: you can lose limbs, your eyesight, you can suffer from kidney failure. But you *can* bring this into remission, you *can* turn back the clock and you *can* get your life back.

I am incredibly grateful to have two fabulous doctors contribute to this book. Firstly, I would like to thank the amazing Dr David Unwin. David and his wife Jen are pioneers in the field of low carb for diabetes. I would urge you to view some of David's work and videos shown at www.dietdoctor.com and his work with www.diabetes.co.uk. Secondly, Dr Ian Lake, another wonderful doctor, has very kindly put together a feature on Type 1 diabetes, a very different disease, but he goes on to show how a low-carb diet can also be of benefit with this type of diabetes. Ian has Type 1 diabetes and has a wonderful blog about running on keto with T1, which you can find at www.type1keto.com.

Best of luck to you all. I am here if you need me. Follow my Facebook page EverydaySugarfree and my recipe website www.everyday sugarfree.co.uk. You can also contact me via my website www. sarahflower.co.uk. It is always a pleasure to hear your stories.

Sarah x

Insulin Resistance and Type 2 Diabetes

HOW DID WE GET HERE?

We are seeing the biggest rise in obesity and Type 2 diabetes we have ever seen. We are now at epidemic levels – at the time of writing, according to www.diabetes.co.uk, it is estimated that over 415 million people worldwide are living with diabetes, and this figure is rising. Between 50 and 70 per cent of our society are obese or overweight. We are now seeing children as young as four years old developing Type 2 diabetes and fatty liver disease. We have an abundance of food, including healthy and fresh food at our disposal, yet we are suffering from more diseases than ever before, including cancer, arthritis and Alzheimer's.

WE DON'T GET IT: WE CUT OUT FAT AND EAT LOTS OF HEALTHY WHOLEGRAINS

If we listen to some health organisations, they will have us believe that we are all eating too much and not exercising enough. If we run with this theory, does it mean that since the early eighties, when obesity started to rise dramatically, that we all suddenly started overeating and being lazy? We were told that fat, particularly saturated fats, cause obesity and heart disease, so we are now consuming a low-fat diet full of man-made oils and margarines, topped off with lots of sugar. We are told to reduce our calorie intake in order to lose weight and, as a result, our supermarkets are awash with low-calorie snacks to tempt us. Statistically, we are now exercising more recreationally than ever before, but we are still getting fat and very sick.

Now let's apply some common sense. If we are getting fat on a low-calorie, low-fat diet, can it really be fat that makes us fat? If we look at how our diet has changed in the last few decades, we will see a large increase in our consumption of sugar and refined carbohydrates. Could these actually be the culprits rather than fat?

We have seen a big rise in the consumption of sugar and carbohydrates since the low-fat revolution, simply because they contain half the calories of fat. When you remove fat from a product, you take away the lovely creaminess we all find irresistible. To make the food more palatable, food manufacturers add sugar. These two factors are what has driven our current diet to be over 70 per cent carbohydrate rich. To understand why this has resulted in us gaining weight, we need to look at how our body deals with sugar and carbohydrates.

Our body takes in sugars and carbohydrates and converts these into glucose – what we are told is our main fuel source. Glucose is quite dangerous when it floods into our blood, so our pancreas releases insulin to help move this glucose into a safe place. We use the liver, muscles and, as a last resort, fat cells for storage. Our liver and muscles are the first port of call; however, due to the high levels of carbohydrates and sugars in our diet, these stores are pretty much always full. The only place left is our fat cells. Now, insulin not only helps push the glucose into our fat cells, it also stops us burning the glucose, effectively locking it away. After all, why would it go to the trouble of storing the glucose if it was then going to burn it?

THE HORMONE EFFECT

Insulin also works in cahoots with a couple of other hormones. One is called ghrelin, known as the hunger hormone, which sits in our stomach and growls at us to feed it. Insulin stimulates this hormone, meaning the more sugar and carbs we eat, the hungrier we get. There is another hormone called leptin, which signals to the brain when we are full. Constant insulin production switches off this leptin response (as does pure fructose), meaning we never feel satisfied and full.

This is a really important fact, especially for those who struggle with overeating. You can see the cycle: people are told that they have to eat less and move more; they want to lose weight, so they opt for low-calorie and low-fat food, which is essentially pure carbohydrates as these are half the calories of fat. But, as soon as they reduce their calories, they get more and more hungry. They are then blamed for being greedy, so they get depressed and their confidence dips to an all-time low, so for comfort as well as a physical necessity, they overeat again.

We also need to look at food addiction. Just like being addicted to alcohol, cigarettes or gambling, we can also be addicted to food. It could be food in general or specific foods, such as sugar or even bread. Food stimulation is all around us, especially junk food. Our high streets are bursting with coffee shops and fast-food restaurants, and every till point, even in our chemists and clothes shops, promotes more food and confectionary. We are not even safe at home, with TV adverts stimulating our hunger. But we were not made to eat constantly; every time we eat something we produce insulin. Is it any wonder that we are suffering now?

It is also worth mentioning that lack of sleep can cause havoc with our hormones and adrenal function. Ghrelin is stimulated, leptin is shut off and we see an imbalance of cortisol, which contributes to adrenal fatigue and our blood sugars become imbalanced. Shift workers are especially prone to weight gain due to all of the above.

We are seeing more doctors now adopting the low-carb advice for diabetics. The doctor in the UK who is really leading the way is Dr David Unwin. He has achieved amazing results for his Type 2 diabetic patients and saves his GP practice thousands of pounds a year in the process. He has achieved these results by listening to his patients and helping them to understand the importance of lifestyle and dietary changes. Here he explains more about the low-carbohydrate, higher-healthy-fat diet for pre-diabetics and Type 2 diabetics.

I am the senior partner of a GP practice in Merseyside. We have been offering a lower-carb diet option to our patients with Type 2 diabetes and pre-diabetes for over four years now, because we believe that for many people with these conditions reducing dietary sugar and starch is a good way to regain control of their health. We were awarded the NHS innovator of the year prize for this work in 2016.

What are carbs (carbohydrates)?
They can be seen as foods either containing sugars or built up from sugars, which form their building blocks. The starches in flour,

potatoes, rice and other grains are examples where largely glucose is concentrated by the plant for storage. When we eat these starches, the process of digestion rapidly breaks them back down into glucose, sometimes in surprisingly large quantities, as predicted by the glycaemic index (hence the low GI diet) and demonstrated below.

FOOD ITEM	G INDEX	SERVE SIZE g	How does each food affect blood glucose compared with one 4g teaspoon of table sugar?	From Unwin et al. It is the glycaemic response to, not the carbohydrate content of food that matters in diabetes. The glycaemic index revisited. Journal of Insulin Resistance Aug 2016
Basmati rice	69	150	10.1	
Potato - white, boiled	96	150	9.1	
French fries baked	64	150	7.5	
Spaghetti - white boiled	39	180	6.6	
Sweetcorn boiled	60	80	4.0	
Frozen peas boiled	51	80	1.3	
Banana	62	120	5.7	
Apple	39	120	2.3	
Wholemeal, small slice	74	30	3.0	
Broccoli	54	80	0.2	Other foods in the very low glycaemic range would be chicken, oily fish, almonds, mushrooms and cheese
Eggs	0	60	0	

How does insulin fit in? And why does eating carbs make you more hungry?

After digestion, the glucose released is rapidly absorbed into the bloodstream – the body knows that high sugar levels are toxic to it, so responds by producing the hormone insulin from the pancreas gland.

One of the functions of insulin is to cause particularly your abdominal fat cells and liver to absorb the glucose to produce fat. The resultant lower glucose level causes you to have hunger or carb cravings and you return to the cookie jar to repeat the cycle, getting fatter in the process.

According to many experts on low-carb diets, including Gary Taubes and the late Dr Atkins, lower insulin levels as a result of reduced carb consumption is the main reason for the effectiveness of low-carb diets in Type 2 diabetes. Over 25 good scientific studies have shown the approach to work well.

They feel that when carbs are restricted and insulin levels go down, the fat isn't 'locked' away in the fat cells anymore and becomes accessible for the body to use as energy, leading to a reduced need for eating.

Also, it's quite possible for the body to become adapted to burning fat as its main fuel over several weeks. Many on the low-carb diet notice they lose belly fat first because of this. Someone with diabetes has a particular problem in metabolising glucose, so the blood-sugar levels after a carby meal stay at toxic high levels, possibly damaging the small blood vessels in the eyes, kidneys and other organs. So burning fat instead of glucose as fuel has obvious advantages.

So it seems to make particular sense for those with Type 2 diabetes to eat far fewer carbs, given that we can live well off other foods such as green vegetables, eggs, meat and fish, nuts and healthy fats. The weight loss that comes with the diet can help many diabetics to avoid medication altogether and feel healthier into the bargain!

Will a diet higher in healthy fats increase my cholesterol level?

Surprisingly, low-carb studies often show the opposite because most of the cholesterol in your blood is manufactured from carbs in your liver and has not come from your diet at all. In clinical practice, I have found significant reductions in triglyceride levels, in addition to improved levels of the 'healthy' HDL cholesterol in people eating fewer carbs but more green veg, full-fat dairy, nuts and eggs.

Many of my patients have commented that the low-carb diet is a lifestyle choice rather than a diet for a few weeks, because of course, going back to the carbs will increase blood-sugar levels again, which in turn stimulates insulin levels, worsening obesity to cause a deterioration once again in diabetic control. Having said that, my wife Jen and I went on the low-carb diet with our patients in January 2013. We have both noticed sustained improvements in our health and have learnt to cook such delicious meals so that we have no intention of going back to our old 'carby' habits!

Dr David Unwin FRCGP, Norwood Surgery, Southport

CALORIES

As we have touched on above, the calories-in, calories-out theory of weight is fundamentally flawed. There are several problems when counting calories to lose weight.

Calories are not equal

Your body processes different types of food differently, even if the calorie count is the same.

For instance, a 330ml can of cola contains approximately 140 calories, half a Mars bar contains 130 calories, 20 almonds contain 140 calories, 400g of broccoli contains 136 calories. If we believe in the calorie theory, all these foods should work in the same way when eaten. Could a female still lose weight if she just ate six Mars bars a day, resulting in consuming 1,560 calories? We also need to consider other factors. A calorie is a unit of energy, and food manufacturers gauge this in a laboratory, testing how the food is burned, but our bodies are individual and don't burn in the same precise way. We are affected by our environment, health, hormones, age, digestion and sleep, to name but a few. The variables are endless.

Metabolism

We have to consider what happens to our metabolism when we restrict calories. We can consume 2,000 calories per day and decide we want to lose weight, so restrict our calories to 1,500 per day. The theory is that our body will continue to burn 2,000 calories a day, meaning a 500-calorie deficit will result in us burning up stored fat. Sounds feasible and it can work in the very short term. However, our body soon adapts to the 1,500 calories and switches to running on 1,500 calories or under. So, in order for you to lose weight, you have to continue to reduce the calories every time you stall. You could attempt to do this by incorporating more exercise into your regime. For instance, approximately 150 calories take 30 minutes of intense exercise to burn, but much depends on the individual's size, age and type of exercise, so it's not an exact science, but ultimately you will become exhausted in your quest to keep up with your ever-declining metabolism. Remember exercise also makes you hungry, something that you may already be struggling with.

I was at a PHC (Public Health Collaboration) seminar and the following information was presented by Dr Jason Fung to show statistically how the calories-in, calories-out (eat less, move more) recommendation is proven to fail.

UK General Practice Database 2004–2014:
• **The probability of achieving normal weight – 0.6 per cent**
• **If morbidly obese – 0.1 per cent**
That is a 99.4 per cent chance of failure, and yet we still follow this advice!

Eighty per cent of people with a 10 per cent weight loss will regain their weight within a year.

Calorie counting

Thirdly, and far more importantly, when we calorie count we start to ignore real food and just focus on the calories. The popularity of low-calorie treats such as 10-cal jelly, Muller Light yoghurts, Special K biscuits, rice cakes, popcorn and Weight Watchers proves our obsession is for low-calorie foods rather than buying food for its nutritional content. What these foods all have in common is not that they are low calorie, but rather high in refined carbohydrates, sugars and artificial sweeteners. You often need a chemistry degree to decipher the ingredients list. Switch back to the role of insulin and we can start to see how low-calorie and low-fat foods can actually make us fat.

I work with many clients suffering from a range of ills caused by insulin resistance, as well as clients with Type 2 diabetes. Many of my clients see their symptoms as individual problems that need solving, giving me a list of issues, wanting me to tick them off as we go. Often, the reason they have come to see me is to help combat weight gain, but as we chat it becomes apparent that aches and pains, tiredness, hormonal issues, high blood pressure, headaches, digestive problems and even allergies are all brought into the consultation. My work involves looking at the client as a whole, trying to work out what has caused each symptom in order to resolve or reverse any problems through dietary and lifestyle changes. Diet can have a dramatic effect on our health. We really are what we eat, and we are starting to see the results of this. Our western diet is full of sugar, carbohydrates, man-made fats and chemical concoctions. As a result, we are seeing dramatic rises in obesity, Type 2 diabetes, fatty liver disease, heart disease, cancer, Alzheimer's, arthritis, sleep problems, hormonal issues, allergies, digestive problems and mental-health issues. The good news is that all of these can be improved just by changing the way you eat, and the earlier you start, the less chance you have of suffering from the above in the first place.

Type 2 diabetes can be reversed by diet, but it does take a willingness to make changes and dedication to stick to them. It is extremely frustrating when I meet with clients who have Type 2 diabetes, especially those who come to me for, what they believe, is an unrelated complaint, and they fail to acknowledge the seriousness of this disease. We are led to believe it simply means taking more medication. Some do not change their diet, as they believe the medication does the work for them. This ignorance is not the fault of the patient but a systematic failure of the health system.

Type 2 diabetes is a lifestyle disease. It is totally man-made. We have seen a dramatic rise in Type 2 diabetes in children, something that has never occurred before. We are in an experimental phase where we are unaware of the consequences of young children developing Type 2 diabetes and how it impacts the rest of their lives.

You can make changes not just for your own health, but also for the health of your family, children and grandchildren.

At first glance, this way of eating could be seen as restrictive, hard work and boring, but you are wrong. I have incorporated many family favourites in this book, giving them all a low-carb makeover. Your plate will be full of a variety of colours and flavours (no more beige food!). Eating real food does take a little more time and preparation, but it is worth it in taste and health.

'This is the new medicine, which is going to take 30 years to be accepted. But as far as your health is concerned, you better accept it today. You haven't got 30 years to wait for medicine to catch up...'
Professor Tim Noakes

2

Type 1 Diabetes

We often refer to Type 2 diabetes as simply diabetes, but we need to make a clarification between Type 1 and Type 2 diabetes as they are very different diseases. Type 1 diabetes is where the pancreas produces little or no insulin; Type 2 diabetes is where the body loses its ability to respond to insulin. This book focuses primarily on Type 2 diabetes; however, I have been lucky enough to meet with Dr Ian Lake. He is a GP locum based in Gloucester. He has had a long-term interest in preventive medicine. Having Type 1 diabetes himself, he adopted a ketogenic lifestyle (see explanation on page 12) three years ago and found it was transformative regarding his health and wellbeing. He is a founder member of the Public Health Collaboration, which is a charity funded entirely by members and dedicated to informing and implementing healthy decisions for better public health. He is also a member of the British Society of Lifestyle Medicine, and a medical advisor to www.diabetes.co.uk – impressive credentials! He kindly agreed to share his expertise and knowledge on Type 1 diabetes.

Type 1 diabetes is a condition that responds well to a low-carbohydrate lifestyle. There is nothing particularly difficult to understand about managing Type 1 in this way. In Type 1 diabetes, the body is unable to produce the hormone insulin. Insulin lowers blood glucose. Glucose is the end result of the digestion of starchy foods (such as bread, potatoes, rice, pasta), which contain a lot of carbohydrate (starch), and is also a sugar found in fruit. Table sugar is half glucose. It can be argued, then, that Type 1 diabetes is a condition of carbohydrate intolerance, so it does not really make much sense to eat carbohydrates, does it?

Thankfully, nature has provided us with types of food other than carbohydrates that are more than adequate for the needs of someone with Type 1 diabetes. These are fat and protein. It is very convenient that fats do not require insulin for them to be metabolised in the body, and they can be eaten without raising blood-glucose levels. Protein does raise glucose levels (glucose can be made from protein), but not at the same rate as carbohydrates. Carbohydrates will cause glucose levels to 'spike', whereas protein causes less spiking, more of a 'low plateau'.

So, if one doesn't need that much insulin when eating a low-carbohydrate diet, can insulin be dispensed with completely? Well, in a word, no. It is always necessary to inject insulin in Type 1 diabetics as it is an essential hormone for life processes. The body needs insulin just to exist. Everyone, diabetic or not, needs insulin. People without Type 1 diabetes simply make their own insulin. And just because you are not eating glucose or carbohydrates doesn't mean that the body goes without. Certain key tissues prefer to use glucose as fuel, so the metabolism has evolved to make this possible even during fasting. Glucose can be made 'in-house' in sufficient quantities by tissues such as the liver (mainly from protein), so that the body does not have to rely on its host to eat it at the right time. Evolution would never have happened if humans had to work it out for themselves! The body has evolved to survive human intellect. So, glucose is present in the blood in the right amount even with low-carbohydrate meals. This means that there is a need for insulin to control this internal production of glucose. Type 1s inject long-acting insulin (basal insulin) for this reason. There are reports in Type 2 diabetes of people stopping insulin. This is a different condition to Type 1. It is dangerous to attempt to stop insulin injections in Type 1. Type 1 diabetes is not yet curable, but controlling it can be easier with low-carbohydrate meals.

The hormone insulin lowers blood glucose by stimulating cells to take it in, or, if they are full of glucose, to convert that glucose to fat. All carbohydrates that are eaten in excess of the body's immediate needs end up as fat, to be stored in times of famine (useful back in the day when supermarkets didn't' exist). Could it be that carbohydrates are addictive (they certainly are) because they provide us with food in the summer months to make us fat to survive the winter? We might be eating carbohydrates out of instinct. Carbohydrates might be addictive to help us to survive. We are, *after all, creatures of the planet. The problem is that with carbohydrates now being readily available throughout the whole year, we might be eating 'for the winter that never comes'.*

SO, HOW DOES 'LOW-CARB' WORK?

It is relatively easy for someone with Type 1 diabetes to inject long-acting (basal) insulin and have a fairly normal blood glucose. If the basal dose is correct and someone skips a meal or two, the glucose levels should be stable. If it isn't, most people adjust their basal insulin to ensure stable glucose levels throughout the day, either with one or typically two injections a day.

The problems begin when large amounts of carbohydrates are eaten with every meal. The idea behind conventional diabetes management is to calculate accurately the amount of carbohydrates in every meal (obviously difficult when eating out) and match this with the correct amount of insulin, injected at exactly the right time (food absorption from the stomach is variable), which then miraculously gets into the blood at exactly the right amount (forget the 30 per cent variation in absorption through the skin) to control the rise of blood glucose and achieve normal glucose levels. The insulin will then ideally stop acting at exactly the right time after a meal to stop the blood glucose from falling too low and cause a hypoglycaemic episode. A number of people achieve this reasonably well, but research shows that the number is just 3 per cent achieving a modest target of control. That would be completely unacceptable to those without diabetes.

But normal blood glucose is achievable on low-carbohydrate diets. Richard Bernstein, a veteran Type 1 (if you haven't heard of him, Google him) goes as far as to say that all Type 1 diabetics have a right to a normal glucose. He should know. He has had Type 1 for 70 years, is still working as a doctor aged 83, and had complications which reversed when he adopted a low-carb diet.

For low-carb diets, the principles are the same as for a conventional guideline diet: estimate the carbohydrate and inject the correct amount of insulin. But the significant difference is that there are very few carbs and so very little extra insulin is needed.

And because of this there are no extreme swings of glucose levels that occur in the majority of those on the guideline diet. So, the practice of low-carbohydrate eating is not that unfamiliar to Type 1s, who have been taught carb counting from diagnosis.

There is good evidence that people who adopt a low-carbohydrate lifestyle in Type 1 diabetes have good glucose control and fewer episodes of hypoglycaemia and ketoacidosis, which are dangerous complications of Type 1 diabetes. There is evidence also that the diet can be sustained in the long term, and that depression eases. Win-win, really.

It all went wrong in diabetes when dietary guidelines were introduced for the non-diabetic population that were so low in fat that they became top-heavy with carbohydrate. To make things worse for Type 1s, the new rapid-acting, 'designer' insulins that were introduced at roughly the same time as the guidelines made dietary freedom a tantalising possibility, and so the diet for people with diabetes became the same as for those without the condition.

People with Type 1 diabetes are currently recommended to eat about 300g of carbohydrates a day, which is typical of the guideline diet (55 per cent of your energy should come from carbs). With the low-carbohydrate diet this is around one-tenth at 30g a day, mainly from sources such as vegetables or berry fruits. And we are talking real food. Food that your grandmother might recognise, fresh, nutritious, unprocessed and unrefined. What every diet should be like.

This is a low-carb or ketogenic lifestyle. It should not be thought of exclusively as a diet. The ketogenic lifestyle combines a healthy low-carbohydrate diet with physical activity, stress reduction and adequate sleep. Both physical activity and sleep have beneficial effects in Type 1 diabetes and they increase the sensitivity of the body to insulin, thereby reducing the amount needed and improving control. Stress reduction seems obvious but can be elusive. Regular physical activity can be in whatever form one wishes. It is probably best, though, to mix both aerobic and anaerobic exercise, such as weight training with cycling, walking or dancing activities.

Ketogenesis means nothing more than the production of chemicals called ketone bodies that are the result of the body using fat for fuel. If there is enough insulin (as described above), this is an entirely natural and healthy state. It is called nutritional ketosis. It is happening all the time in all of us, diabetes or not. When you are asleep and not eating, the body fuels itself on fat. It just uses the fat stored from the previous day's excesses. In fact, when one looks at the biochemistry, the body seems to prefer fat over glucose for most of its metabolism.

There is little need to worry about reducing carbohydrates and replacing them with fat. Fat is twice as energy dense as carbohydrates, so in reality not much is needed. If it comes from sources such as butter, olive oil and fish, with meat from pasture-fed animals (a better fat profile) there is little to be concerned about. The idea that saturated fat is harmful to health has been revised by many national bodies. 60 per cent of the brain is fat, and healthy fats such as those mentioned here contain favourable ratios of fats considered ideal for maintaining a healthy brain. Not all fat in the body is used for the purposes of providing energy. A large amount is 'structural' fat in that it is a vital constituent of cell membranes in all tissues of the body. Other fats have anti-inflammatory properties and are vital in the maintenance of health. This is especially true of polyunsaturated fats. Fat is important for health in general, but that does not mean that the diet needs to be top-heavy in fat. True, a diet with about three-quarters of energy coming from fat keeps glucose levels stable, and this is desirable, but a healthy body also needs a supply of nutrients. So, don't forget protein and plants, which contain a wider range of nutrients than fat and are essential for robust health. Most importantly, have fun.

Dr Ian Lake

If you want to find out more about Dr Lake's work, he has a fascinating blog on running and Type 1 diabetes, which can be found at www.type1keto.com, primarily showing that carbohydrates are not essential in Type 1 diabetes, and demonstrating that 'extreme diabetes' is not about eliminating carbs and fasting, but rather following conventional advice

3
....

Sugars and Fats

We all need to be cutting our sugar consumption dramatically. In 2015, the World Health Organization set new guidelines. It recommended everyone reduce their daily intake of free sugars (see below) to less than 10 per cent of their total energy intake. A further reduction to below 5 per cent, or roughly 25g (6 teaspoons) per day for adults, would provide additional health benefits. Pour this into a glass and you can see it is quite a substantial amount, but shockingly, some low-fat yoghurt desserts can contain more than the maximum set per day. Looking at the amount of sugar in our food, is it easy to see why we are on average consuming 30–40 teaspoons per day!

Free sugars refer to monosaccharides (such as glucose and fructose) and disaccharides (such as sucrose or table sugar) added to foods and drinks by the manufacturer, cook or consumer, and sugars naturally present in honey, syrups, fruit juices and fruit juice concentrates.

'We have solid evidence that keeping intake of free sugars to less than 10% of total energy intake reduces the risk of overweight, obesity and tooth decay,' says Dr Francesco Branca, Director of WHO's Department of Nutrition for Health and Development. 'Making policy changes to support this will be key if countries are to live up to their commitments to reduce the burden of non-communicable diseases.'

But do we really understand sugar? Let's get down to absolute basics.

- Sugar is made up of 50 per cent glucose and 50 per cent fructose, but has no nutrient value at all and, despite what some may claim, it is not needed by the body at all. You could live quite happily without **any** added sugar.
- There are many names for sugar – maple syrup, honey, molasses, brown sugar, agave syrup, high-fructose corn syrup, barley malt, cane sugar, dextran, sucrose, maltose, maltodextrin, ethyl maltol,

lactose, and the list goes on. These all affect the body in the same way, so don't be fooled.

- Carbohydrates (think flour, pasta, bread, sugar, vegetables, beans, grains and starchy foods such as potatoes) get converted into glucose, providing us with energy. However, we are consuming more than we have ever eaten in our existence, and it is this excess consumption that is so detrimental to our health. Our body can run extremely well on fat, protein and limited carbohydrates. Limiting sugars and carbohydrates can greatly reduce a number of ills.
- Fructose is now deemed to be the most damaging sugar form, and is linked to non-alcoholic fatty liver disease (NAFLD) and heart disease. Fructose also interferes with our leptin response and is shown to lay down more visceral fat (the fat around your vital organs).
- Fructose is also found in fruit. Eating a whole fruit means that you are also eating some fibre, which slows down the digestion of the fructose. However, drink your fruit in fruit juice and you have no fibre, therefore a high concentration of fructose floods the liver. Suddenly, your fresh orange juice in the morning contains more sugar than a glass of cola. It is also interesting that studies have shown that when you drink pure fructose, it turns off your leptin response, meaning you don't get the signal to tell you when you are full.

There is a very long list of health complaints that experts believe stem from sugar. It is a very scary list and, if you are like me, it is enough to focus the mind and dig deep to maintain a sugar-free lifestyle.

HEALTH COMPLAINTS THAT EXPERTS BELIEVE STEM FROM SUGAR

This is not a definitive list, but just the tip of the iceberg:

Obesity
Type 2 diabetes
Metabolic syndrome
Alzheimer's
Arthritis
Autoimmune disease

Gout
Fatty liver disease
Heart disease
Depression
Hyperactivity
Anxiety
Insomnia
Inflammation
Inability to concentrate
High blood pressure
High cholesterol
Low immune system
Cancer
Ageing
Tooth decay
Learning difficulties
Candida
Thrush
Gallstones
Appendicitis
Haemorrhoids
Varicose veins
Osteoporosis
Food intolerances
PMS (pre-menstrual syndrome)
PCOS (polycystic ovary syndrome)
Mood swings

WHAT DO WE NEED TO AVOID?

Avoiding added sugar and foods high in fructose is an absolute must. You will find this in a variety of guises on food labels, so be vigilant. You also need to be aware of free sugars – these are the naturally occurring ones or those added to the food's supposedly natural state. Think of fruit juices, syrups and honeys. It is a minefield, but the simple thing is to read the labels and to try as much as possible to make your own food from scratch.

You also need to be aware of the foods that convert to glucose once consumed. Carbohydrates and starches not only add to your daily sugar load, but also spike insulin and increase food cravings, so to be successful when going sugar free, you really need to watch your carbohydrate intake and limit it to 20–30g per day for active health changes.

'People are fed by the food industry, which pays no attention to health, and treated by the health industry which pays no attention to food.'

Wendell Berry, American novelist and activist/environmentalist

READ THE LABEL

Labelling is not as straightforward as it should be, with manufacturers trying to confuse us. You need a calculator to work out correct serving sizes to give you the amount of sugar per gram and to then convert into teaspoons. When you look at the amount of sugar per teaspoon it is very scary.

Here are some names you need to avoid:

Sucrose, Fructose, High-fructose corn syrup, Barley malt, Dextrose, Maltose, Agave nectar, Beet sugar, Cane juice, Turbinado sugar, Caramel, Carob syrup, Corn syrup, Date sugar, Dextrin, Evaporated cane juice, Fruit juice, Grape juice, Diastase, Glucose, Maltol, Palm sugar, Monoglycerides, Refiners syrup, Mannose, Oligofructose, Tapioca syrup, Maple syrup, Treacle, Saccharose, Molasses, Coconut sugar, Polydextrose, Glycerine, Yakon, Dextran, Diastatic malt powder, Sorghum, Ethyl maltol, Galactose, Golden syrup, Honey, Inverted sugar, Lactose, Maltodextrin, Muscovado sugar, Oat syrup, Avena sativa, Panela, Panocha, Crystalline fructose.

ARTIFICIAL SWEETENERS

I avoid artificial sweeteners as I have read too many papers linking their use to mental-health problems and health complaints. There is now mounting evidence to show that artificial sweeteners are highly addictive, increase your sugar cravings and continue to lead to obesity. They can also contribute to insulin resistance and diabetes, and have been linked to headaches, hypertension, mental-health issues, anxiety and even seizures.

Many of my clients are addicted to sugar-free/diet fizzy drinks. It is one of the first things we have to eliminate from their diet in order to move ahead to better health and weight loss.

NATURAL SWEETENERS

There is a lot of misinformation regarding sugar free. Some people opt to be free of refined sugar, instead opting for maple syrup, agave or honey. However, a word of warning. You are still taking in sugars in the form of glucose and, most worryingly, fructose. Your body metabolises all sugars in the same way, whether they are from refined or natural sources, so really, you are just taking a sideways step. You will also continue to crave sweet foods, so it will make your sugar-free journey so much harder. Agave contains over 90 per cent fructose.

One of the main objectives of this book is to help you train your palate off sugar and sweet cravings, so that you don't want to swap one sugar for another alternative. By all means use the natural sweeteners as a transition towards sugar free, but gradually reduce your intake of sweeteners as your palate changes. I hardly use any natural sweeteners in food now, as I tend to find it sweet enough.

RECOMMENDED SWEETENERS

The three sugar alternatives I would recommend (stevia, xylitol and erythritol) are fructose free, meaning they have very little adverse impact on health. Although some of the recipes in this book include these sweeteners, I must emphasise that the key is to have these as treats to help you in the transition phase of becoming sugar free and not to overdo the sweet hits.

Stevia is a wild plant from the subtropical forest in North East Paraguay. The leaves of stevia contain glycosides, of which sweetening power is between 250 and 400 times their equivalent in sugar. Stevia contains no calories and no carbohydrates. It does not raise blood sugar or stimulate an insulin response, so for many, it is the preferred choice as it is completely natural.

However, stevia (the cheapest of all three) is very sweet and does have a strange aftertaste, which is hard to control. I have found liquid stevia has less of an aftertaste, but it is really down to trial and error and depends on the brand you use. I use SweetLeaf stevia drops as they have the least 'aftertaste'. I buy these from Amazon, but they are becoming more available in UK stores.

Stevia is very hard to gauge in recipes as it is very much down to personal taste, brand and your sensitivity to the aftertaste. If you are new to it, you may prefer to use xylitol or erythritol, but if you are a fan of stevia, you can still follow my recipes, but tweak the stevia quantities to suit your own taste.

Xylitol looks just like sugar. Xylitol may sound slightly odd, but the word is derived from the Greek word for wood 'xyl', as in xylophone, because the natural sugar alternative was first discovered in birch wood. Xylitol has now been found in a host of other plants and fruits, such as sweetcorn and plums, but is still largely extracted from birch and beech wood in Europe today.

Xylitol looks and tastes just like regular granulated sugar, but it has a host of benefits. It has 40 per cent fewer calories than normal sugar and less than 50 per cent of the available carbohydrates (those that are utilised by your body), but it does contain carbohydrates, and therefore does stimulate an insulin response, so it is not suitable for everyone.

Xylitol can have a laxative effect in some people if eaten to excess. The laxative effect is caused because xylitol attracts water to it. This effect is different from person to person and can change as your body gets use to xylitol. The lower your body weight, the less xylitol it takes to cause the effect, so children can be more affected. As a general rule, daily consumption should be limited to 5–10g per 10kg of body weight (adults and children alike).

You also need to keep xylitol, or any food made with it, well clear of dogs. As with grapes and chocolates, dogs metabolise xylitol quite differently from humans and it can be very dangerous for them, even in small amounts. Don't be tempted to give your dog anything with xylitol in, no matter how small.

The UK's leading brand of xylitol is Total Sweet (www.totalsweet.co.uk). It is made from sustainable European birch and beech wood, and is available in most supermarkets.

Erythritol is found in blends from companies such as Natvia and Surkin. Just like xylitol, this is a sugar alcohol known as a poll, which is found in grapes and pears. Erythritol can be bought in the form of icing sugar, granulated sugar and even brown sugar. Again, use this as a direct replacement in recipes, but be aware that manufacturers often add stevia to these blends as erythritol on its own is not so sweet, so you may still detect a slight aftertaste.

Unlike other sugar-free, low-calorie substitutes like xylitol, erythritol contains zero calories. Erythritol does not affect blood sugar or insulin levels during or after consumption, making it safe for diabetics and for those following a LCHF diet.

Unlike other sugar alcohols such as xylitol, maltitol and isomalt, erythritol is well absorbed from the digestive tract, passed into the urine and eliminated from the body, so it does not have a laxative side effect.

OTHER NATURAL SUGARS

Fructose

My concern about all sugars, including natural sugars and fruit, is based on the glucose and fructose content. Most of us are familiar with the basics of glucose and know it is associated with raising insulin and its role in diabetes. We may not, however, be so familiar with the negative effects of fructose.

- Fructose has been shown to increase the production of endogenous AGEs (advanced glycation end products), which have been linked to age-related and degenerative disorders. Those with high blood sugars also appear to produce more AGEs.
- Fructose gets pushed into our liver and converted to fats, which can store in the liver, attributing to non-alcoholic fatty liver disease, as

well as being pushed into our adipose tissue contributing to obesity and related conditions.

- It also gets pushed into our blood as triglycerides, as well as raising our small LDL particles and oxidised LDL.
- Fructose can increase whole body inflammation and the risk of oxidative damage in our cells. It also increases uric acid production, which can lead to high blood pressure, gout and kidney stones.
- Fructose is also very addictive and stimulates the hormone ghrelin, which growls at us to eat more and can shut off our leptin response (the hormone that tells our brain when we are full).
- It also has a detrimental effect on our looks, as it interferes with collagen production, decreasing our skin elasticity and increasing our risk of wrinkles.
- Your bowel health can be affected. Bad bacteria feed off of the sugars in your diet, particularly fructose. Poor bowel health not only affects your digestion and bowel habits but also lowers your immune system and can increase your risk of tumours. Poor bowel health also impacts on how your body deals with cholesterol. My advice is to avoid anything high in fructose.

Coconut sugar

You many think coconut sugar comes from coconuts, but it is really palm sugar. As with all sugars, my concern is the glucose and fructose content. Coconut sugar contains inulin, which helps reduce/slow the absorption of glucose, but before we get too excited, unlike stevia, xylitol and erythritol, coconut sugar still causes a rise in blood sugars. Coconut sugar is made up of sucrose, glucose and fructose. Sucrose is 50 per cent glucose and fructose, so if we add everything together, coconut sugar contains 40–50 per cent fructose. This is pretty much the same as standard sugar. It is popular as it contains a lot of nutrients, which is positive, but you can get these nutrients from other foods without the associated high levels of fructose and glucose.

Maple syrup

Many celebrity chefs are now using maple syrup instead of sugar, but I see this as a sideways step. Yes, maple syrup is natural, but your body still breaks it down in the same way as sugar, honey, brown sugar or whatever sweet thing you may eat. Just like coconut sugar, it does contain more nutrients than refined sugar, but that does not make it a good choice. We need to be more concerned about the glucose and fructose content. Maple syrup is almost 100 per cent sucrose which, just like table sugar, is made up of 50 per cent glucose and 50 per cent fructose. It will spike your blood sugar in exactly the same way as refined sugar.

Agave syrup

Another sideways step. It got a health push because it was a lower GI than refined sugar, meaning it does not cause so much of a blood spike. However, we are forgetting the damaging effects of fructose. Agave syrup contains the most fructose of any of the 'natural' sugar replacements, with up to 97 per cent fructose. This is actually higher than high-fructose corn syrup!

Dates

These are used a lot to help sweeten desserts and baked goods. Date-based bars are advocated as healthy because they contain no refined sugar, or no added sugar, but don't be fooled, as these are naturally packed with sugar and will raise blood sugars and flood your liver with fructose in exactly the same way.

Fruit

Eat whole fruits rather than drinking fruit juices or concentrates. I tend to opt for berries, as these are lower in fructose. Fill up with nutritious vegetables and only use whole fruits when needed. If you like juices or smoothies, opt for vegetable juices that contain only a very small amount of fruit. This way you will gain the essential nutrients and antioxidants but limit your consumption of damaging fructose.

Fat

We have been demonising fat since the late 1970s. The research behind the low-fat revolution is actually fundamentally flawed. Dr Ancel Keys wanted to demonstrate that heart disease was caused by saturated fat. He couldn't quite prove his theory, so rather than hold his hands up and admit he might be wrong, he effectively ignored the data that disproved his theory. Since then we have lived in fear of fat. Although we eat less fat than ever before, obesity, diabetes, heart disease, cancer and Alzheimer's are all increasing rapidly. If we listen to the latest health advice, we are getting fat because we eat too much and don't exercise enough. Did we all suddenly become greedy and lazy since the late 1970s? I think not.

All foods containing fat also contain saturated fat, polyunsaturated fat and monounsaturated fat, and the ratios may surprise you. I recently went to a conference where Zoe Harcombe, a leading food researcher (www.zoeharcombe.com), shocked the audience when she demonstrated that skimmed milk contains more saturated fat than unsaturated. Omega 3-rich mackerel contains 1.5 times more saturated fat than a sirloin steak, and 1 tablespoon of olive oil could contain more saturated fat than a pork chop weighing 100g.

We fear saturated fat, but it is absolutely essential for our health, brain, nerves and lungs, right through to our heart and joint health. We need fat to absorb our fat-soluble vitamins such as vitamins A, E, D and K. Healthy, natural fats do not make you fat; fat keeps us feeling fuller for longer. Once we restrict our carbohydrates and insulin spikes, fat becomes our main fuel source. We become fat burners instead of sugar burners.

We have demonised natural fats while embracing man-made polyunsaturated fats and oils (and don't get me started on trans fats!). These oils go rancid and toxic incredibly quickly, especially when exposed to heat, light and oxygen. They cause havoc in our body, attacking every organ and our cell membranes, including our red blood cells and even our DNA. We need to opt for more natural, stable oils such as extra-virgin olive oil or avocado oil, and try to gain an equal balance between omega-3 and omega-6 consumption. Excessive consumption of omega-6 causes whole body inflammation (omega-6 fats are pro-inflammatory, whereas omega-3 fats are anti-inflammatory). Add this to our diet of excessive refined carbohydrates and sugars and you start to have an understanding of why we are experiencing major health problems.

WHAT ABOUT CHOLESTEROL?

Our fear of fat centres on saturated fats and the dreaded cholesterol. Saturated fat does not cause heart disease. It is far more complicated. In fact, we only get 20 per cent of our cholesterol from food. Cholesterol is needed for almost every function in the human body, from nerve and brain function to digestion and cell health. It is present in every cell membrane, helping to maintain structure and stability, and also helps repair cells and tissues. Our bodies produce up to 1g of cholesterol a day to help synthesise hormones, assisting in the production of hormones such as oestrogen, progesterone, testosterone and cortisol. Cholesterol is also vital for brain function; in fact 60 per cent of our brain is made up of fat and cholesterol. It also helps us to digest fat and convert sunlight into vitamin D, which in turn helps to lower blood pressure.

Old low-fat guidelines would have led you to believe that increased LDL levels indicate you are consuming too much saturated fats and need to opt for a better diet. LDL particles can be large or small, with the small, oxidised ones linked to the damage, including inflammation in the arteries. However, when you consume saturated fats, this changes the small LDL particles into large ones, in effect, making them safe. The role of cholesterol is to provide structure and support for cell walls, so an increase in LDL can be due to the body trying to repair damaged endothelial cell walls. Increased levels could also be due to the body being unable to break down excess cholesterol (familial hypercholesterolemia), which affects 1 in every 500. The liver also produces more cholesterol when we are stressed or suffering from ill health and inflammation, which goes hand in hand with the increase in cortisol hormone. Oxidised small LDL particles are also caused by free radicals. Therefore a diet rich in antioxidants such as blueberries, pecans and walnuts, as well as a diet avoiding processed foods, particularly those packed with trans fats, is one of the best ways to keep your heart healthy.

A recent study published in the *BMJ Open Journal* found that 92 per cent of elderly people with high cholesterol lived longer. The book *The Great Cholesterol Con* by Dr Malcolm Kendrick, makes fascinating reading, with reference to many studies showing that reducing your cholesterol may in fact increase your risk of cardiovascular disease. There are other factors that cause us to have heart disease, such as the negative role of our consumption of inflammatory man-made oils, what causes endothelial damage, and the role of triglycerides. Triglycerides are a fat found in the food we eat but are also produced by the liver. They are stored in the liver or fat cells but can also be found travelling in our blood. High triglycerides contribute to heart disease, Type 2 diabetes and fatty liver disease. Alcohol consumption and some medications such as beta blockers can also raise triglyceride levels.

4

Getting Started

Deciding to take control of your health is the hardest step; the rest is easy. The key is to plan ahead and to gain as much knowledge as possible, as this will help motivate and inspire you to stick to a healthier way of eating. Remember, this is not a short-term diet, this is a long-term way of eating for optimum health.

PREPARE, PREPARE, PREPARE

Before you get started, you need to prepare. The more time you put into the preparation, the easier you will find the transition to a low-carb way of eating. Take time to read the chapters in this book, especially the food lists and store-cupboard recommendations.

EMPOWERMENT: KNOWLEDGE IS POWER

Whenever I have worked with clients to change their diet in quite a radical way, I have always had far better results when the client understands why we are making the changes. When things get tough, it is a really good idea to focus on why you are doing this, the positives for you and your family, and envisage the end results. Spend time reading, viewing lectures on YouTube or subscribing to experts' Facebook pages. Knowledge is power.

FURTHER READING

This is a recipe book and I wanted to keep it light and easy to follow, but I thoroughly recommend further reading and increasing your knowledge of why we should eliminate sugar, fructose and refined, high carbohydrates from our diet. I share lots of information on my Facebook page and website – EverydaySugarFree. There is a whole host of information available on the internet. Please refer to the reference section at the back of this book for more information to help empower you and your family.

'I am definitely not the same person I was when this year started'

'Etienne was well on the road to ill health. A Type 2 diabetic dependant on insulin, he was also on a wide range of medications for high blood pressure and high cholesterol which, despite his medication, was still high.

'When Etienne started banting [another term for the LCHF lifestyle], he was not sleeping well, could not get out of bed in the mornings and was always tired. He and his wife started banting in July 2016. Within nine months his cholesterol dropped from 7.8 to 2.8; his blood sugar down from 13 to 5.2; and his weight dropped from 140kg to 114kg. At the time of writing he has another 15kg to lose, but by September 2017, Etienne was off all his medication. His wife also lost weight, dropping from 95kg to 79kg. They have no problem getting up early and often have a quick cycle before work. They even compete in local cycling events. Best of all, they have got their life back.'

South African Banting Coach, Amanda Strydom

PREP YOUR KITCHEN

It is estimated that almost 90 per cent of supermarket foods contain sugar, which is a daunting prospect for families about to embark on a sugar-free journey. Spend time going through your cupboards and preparing them for your new way of eating. Read the labels of your favourite foods and try to keep a tally on what you consume per day. There are some apps available now to help you with this, such as MyFitnessPro. You may also find some keto and LCHF apps that can help. I like the KetoDiet app. You will also find great inspiration from downloading a magazine from South Africa called *Lose It!*.

Remember, your essential store cupboard list will be a fair bit smaller, as most processed foods, including condiments, contain high levels of sugar. You may want to have a look at the recipes in The Pantry (p239–252) to whizz up everyday essentials you and your family need, such as tomato sauce, spice blends and jams.

FIZZY DRINKS

Many of my clients, particularly those who have been on low-calorie diets, are addicted to sugar-free, diet soft drinks. Coca-Cola is the one that most people struggle to eliminate. I cannot stress enough how important it is for you to knock artificial sweeteners on the head when following a sugar-free diet. I know that may sound odd, but research has found that those who are consuming artificial sweeteners, particularly in fizzy drinks, have a higher risk of diabetes and related illnesses, as well as an inability to lose weight.

There really is no easy way to ease yourself off the addiction. You just have to stop and go through the withdrawal. This can be tough, as it really is cold turkey, but don't give in. Within a week you will feel so much better. Initially you may suffer from fatigue, irritability, maybe even flu-like symptoms, but stick with it – I promise it will be worth it in the end.

Replace fizzy drinks with sparkling water infused with fruit, herbal teas or coconut water. There is a new sugar-free drinks brand on the market called Ugly (www.uglydrinks.com). Their drinks are available in lemon and lime, and grapefruit and pineapple flavours. They are free from sweeteners and sugar and are naturally flavoured.

EMOTION

We all have an emotional connection with food. Think about your childhood. Most of us were given treats as a reward for good behaviour; we would have treats and sugary food to celebrate; we would be offered sweets and treats to help when we were down, poorly or suffering our first broken heart. Our emotions are intrinsically linked with how we are feeling and our social life, so breaking free of this hold can be a challenge.

Think about how your emotions affect your eating habits. Are you an emotional eater, grabbing the nearest chocolate bar when you are feeling down? Do you eat through boredom? Do you like to celebrate with your friends and feel the diet restriction could inhibit your social life? Think about these things and try to formulate a plan of how you will deal with different situations.

- **Emotional eating:** The secret here is to plan ahead and ensure your fridge and store cupboard are well stocked for such an eventuality. I am an emotional eater. I crave chocolate when I am really low and dealing with too much stress. My secret is always to have some dark chocolate (I now eat 100 per cent dark chocolate), chia seeds and cacao powder in my store cupboard, as well as cream, avocado and berries in my fridge. Within minutes I can have a chocolate mousse, raspberries and cream, or a chocolate chia pudding. If I can't wait 5 minutes, I'll have a square of dark chocolate.
- **Social life:** This depends very much on what you are doing and planning, but eating out is not really a problem as long as you are clever with your menu choices. If you are booking a restaurant in advance, just give them a call and explain you are sugar free and low carb. As you progress on this way of eating, you will get adapt at swapping to make a meal suit your low-carb, sugar-free diet. Most restaurants I have been to, even on an impromptu visit, are happy to accommodate. Most menus can be adapted quite easily, for example, swapping chips for extra salad, opting for a burger without the bun, a carvery without the roast potatoes, or an all-day breakfast without the beans, hash browns, etc., but filling up on extra bacon and eggs. I truly believe we should keep asking for sugar-free options when we are out, as this will gradually filter through to create change. It was not that many years ago when you would struggle to get anything gluten free, and now gluten-free options are in every coffee shop and restaurant.
- **Boredom:** Boredom can manifest itself as hunger, but you need to be aware of this. Some people find drinking a glass of water can help (dehydration can also be confused with hunger pangs). If you eat through boredom, think of ways to distract yourself or to keep yourself busy. Eating high-fat foods is a great way to curb hunger pangs.
- **Conscious eating:** Have you ever sat in front of the TV and consumed a whole pot of ice cream or a jumbo packet of crisps and

had no recollection of doing so? Paul McKenna did an experiment on one of his TV programmes on conscious eating. Cinema goers were given a box of popcorn before they were seated. When they came out of the cinema, all the boxes were empty. They were asked if they wanted more popcorn and some said yes. They then realised the popcorn was stale, yet when watching the film, they did not notice.

It is also interesting to note that those families who eat in front of the TV tend to be more prone to weight gain. This is due to them ignoring the 'feeling full' response as they are too busy concentrating on what is on the TV. Do you eat unconsciously? If so, plan your snacks before you sit down in front of the TV.

'Fitness is 20% exercise and 80% nutrition. You can't outrun a bad diet.'

Dr Aseem Malhotra, award-winning cardiologist and author of *The Pioppi Diet*

5

Good and Bad Foods

Please read this chapter very carefully as it contains everything you need to know about the foods you can eat, as well as those you can't.

DIETARY RECOMMENDATIONS

For faster weight loss, choose only from the Unlimited Foods list. The Occasional Foods list can be used every so often, but the more you eat from this list, the slower your weight loss will be. The Foods You Must Not Eat list is a complete no-no. And remeber, you should have no more that 20–30g of carbs per day.

'Every time you eat or drink, you are either feeding disease or fighting it.'

Heather Morgan, MS, NLC

UNLIMITED FOODS

Just as the title implies, the following list shows all the foods you can eat. These foods contain less than 5g of carbohydrates per 100g, meaning they are very low carb. Dairy, meat, eggs and fish are staple foods, along with (non-starchy) vegetables. The joy of this way of eating is feeling satisfied after eating, and unlike a low-calorie/low-fat diet, you are not fighting hunger.

   Remember, although these foods are deemed unlimited, if you find you are not losing weight or your blood sugars are not coming down, you may need to start calculating your carbohydrates to ensure you are consuming no more than 20–30g per day. The rule of thumb is to eat only when hungry and stop when full.

All eggs

All meats, poultry and game
Opt for quality meats, ideally organic/grass-fed if you can afford to do so.
- Including all-natural cured meats (such as bacon, pancetta and Parma ham).
- All natural and cured sausages (such as salami and chorizo). Ensure all sausages are free from grains and as natural as possible.
- All offal.

Fish
- Oily fish rich in omega-3, such as salmon, tuna, mackerel, pilchards, trout and haddock.
- All seafood (except swordfish and tilefish because of the high mercury content).

Broths
- Bone broth
- Chicken broth
- Vegetable broth

Dairy products
It is really important to always opt for full-fat/whole dairy products. If you can, choose organic. Be aware of the carbohydrate count of dairy (lactose is a form of sugar); it can add up quite quickly, especially if you add milk to tea or coffee. Some women may find dairy hinders weight loss, especially those that are hormonal or pre-menopausal.
- Full-fat milk
- Full-fat cottage cheese
- Full-fat cream cheese
- All soft cheeses (but not processed commercial cheese spreads such as Dairylea)
- All hard cheeses
- Full-fat single, double and extra-thick cream
- Butter
- Full-fat natural Greek yoghurt

Oils and fats
- Butter
- Coconut oil
- Duck/goose fat
- Ghee
- Lard
- Avocado oil
- Macadamia oil
- Good-quality olive oil
- Good-quality flax oil

Flavourings and condiments
- All flavourings and condiments are okay, provided they do not contain sugars and preservatives or vegetable (seed) oils (read the labels!).
- Mayonnaise, full fat only (not from seed oils)
- Tomato ketchup (homemade and sugar free)
- Salt is essential, especially if you start to feel nauseous or suffer from headaches

Flours and thickeners
- Baking powder
- Ground almonds
- Almond flour
- Nut flours (hazelnut, brazil nut, walnut)
- Seed flours (flax seed, sunflower)
- Whey protein
- Xanthan gum
- Psyllium husk
- Gelatine

Nuts and seeds
- Almonds (including almond flour and ground almonds)
- Brazil nuts
- Chia seeds
- Coconut (including coconut flour)
- Flaxseeds
- Hazelnuts

- Macadamia nuts
- Pecan nuts
- Pine nuts
- Pumpkin seeds
- Pure nut butters (but not peanut butter)
- Sunflower seeds
- Walnuts

Sweeteners
- Erythritol granules (Natvia or Sukrin brands are good in the UK)
- Stevia powder or liquids
- Xylitol granules (called Total Sweet and available in supermarkets)

Vegetables
- All green leafy vegetables and salad leaves (spinach, cabbage, lettuces)
- Any other vegetables grown above the ground (except butternut)
- Asparagus
- Aubergines
- Avocados
- Broccoli
- Brussels sprouts
- Cabbage
- Cauliflower
- Celery
- Courgettes
- Kale
- Mushrooms
- Olives
- Onions
- Peppers
- Pumpkin
- Radishes
- Sauerkraut
- Spring onions
- Tomatoes (including tinned and pure tomato purée)

Chocolate
- Dark chocolate (at least 85% cocoa or cacao content)
- Sugar-free cocoa or cacao

Herbs and spices
Unlimited herbs and spices, but read the labels as a lot of spice blends can contain sugar and grain

Drinks and beverages
- Tea and coffee are fine as long as you are not affected by caffeine – watch the milk as the lactose can add up your carb count
- Water and sparkling water
- There are more and more natural, sugar-free drinks coming on to the market, but be sure to read the labels for hidden sugars and artificial sweeteners. I like Ugly Drinks (www.uglydrinks.com)

OCCASIONAL FOODS
The foods listed here really are occasional treats. The more you dip into this list, the slower your progress will be. These foods contain up to 25g per 100g of carbohydrates. I have stated rough guides of carbohydrate counts in the list below. This list should not be followed daily until your blood sugar is stable and you have achieved adequate weight loss. It is more for those wanting to maintain their weight rather than those actively seeking to lose weight or bring Type 2 diabetes into remission.

Fruits (carbohydrate content per 50g)
Remember to view fruit as natures candy!
- Apples (6.5g)
- Apricots, fresh (6.5g)
- Bananas (9.4g)
- Blackberries (4.3g)
- Blueberries (6.1g)

- Cherries, fresh (4.7g)
- Figs, fresh (6.8g)
- Gooseberries (6g)
- Grapes (7.4g)
- Guavas (7.7g)
- Kiwi fruits (6.5g)
- Lemons (7g)
- Mangos, fresh (6.8g)
- Nectarines (5.2g)
- Oranges (4.6g)
- Papaya (4.6g)
- Peaches (4.3g)
- Pears (7.2g)
- Pineapple (6.1g)
- Plums (5.5g)
- Raspberries (2.6g)
- Strawberries (3g)
- Watermelon (3g)

Nuts
- Cashew nuts, raw (30g per 100g)
- Chestnuts, raw (28g per 100g)

Vegetables (carbohydrate content per 100g)
- Artichoke (14.3g)
- Beetroot (8g)
- Butternut (10.2g)
- Carrots (6.4g)
- Leek (12.4g)
- Parsnips (13g)
- Sweet potatoes (17.4g)

EATING TO BEAT TYPE 2 DIABETES

FOODS YOU MUST NOT EAT

This is a list of banned foods. Be sure to read all ingredients lists to ensure you are not inadvertently taking in any of the banned foods. This way of eating is all about eating real food and avoiding any processed/junk foods.

Baked goods
- Including cakes, biscuits, crackers and confectionary, as they all contain grains and sugar
- All products made with flours from grains (such as wheat flour, cornflour, rye flour, barley flour, pea flour, rice flour, rice cakes)

Please note that gluten-free products are not grain free. Most gluten-free products contain grains in the form of rice as well as starches such as potato starch, all of which are high in carbohydrates. Remember, all baked goods need to be made from scratch using fresh LCHF ingredients (see pp43-44).

Bread
- All forms of bread, including gluten free.

Remember, you can make your own bread from scratch using LCHF ingredients (see pp43-44)

All grains, pseudograins and corns
- Wheat, oats, barley, rye, amaranth, quinoa, spelt, buckwheat, millet, cornflower, rice, couscous, teff, sorghum, brans, popcorn, polenta, corn thins, maize

All beans and pulses (dried or canned)
- Butter beans
- Cannellini beans
- Chickpeas
- Haricot beans
- Lentils
- Red kidney beans
- Split peas

'Breaded' and battered foods
- Such as processed chicken nuggets, battered fish, breaded ham.

Breakfast cereals
- Avoid all breakfast cereals, even if the label states no added sugar. This includes muesli and granola

Avoid all pastas, noodles and rice
This includes all forms of rice, including rice flours; and all pasta, including vegetable and gluten-free pasta.

Thickening agents
- Gravy powder, maize starch, cornflour or stock cubes, as these contain grains and sugar. Instead, opt for xanthium gum, arrowroot or nut flours to thicken. Use bone broth instead of stock cubes

Beverages
- Beer
- Cider
- Fizzy drinks (sodas) of any description other than carbonated water
- Lite, zero, diet drinks of any description
- Cordials

Dairy/Dairy-related
- Cheese spreads
- Commercial spreads
- Coffee creamers
- Commercial almond milk
- Condensed milk
- Reduced-fat cow's milk
- Rice milk
- Soya milk
- Ice cream

Seed oils and commercial oils
- All types of margarine
- Canola oil
- Corn oil

- Cottonseed oil
- Grapeseed oil
- Hydrogenated or partially hydrogenated oils
- Rapeseed oil
- Safflower oil
- Sunflower oil
- Vegetable fats

Chocolate
- All commercial chocolate and confectionary, except for pure dark chocolate (at least 85% cacao content)

Commercial sauces, marinades and salad dressings
These include all commercial sauces, such as tomato ketchup, brown sauce and salad creams. Be aware that most salad dressings contain sugars and seed oils, so it's best to make your own.

Fruits and vegetables
- Fruit juice of any kind
- Vegetable juices (other than homemade using vegetables from the Unlimited Foods list)
- Potatoes (regular)

Meat
- All unfermented soya (vegetarian 'protein')
- Meats cured with excessive sugar
- Vienna sausages, luncheon meats

General
- All fast foods
- All low-fat foods
- All processed foods
- Any food with added sugar (read the label for hidden sugars such as dextrose, glucose, fruit syrups and fruit concentrates)

Sweeteners
- Agave
- Artificial sweeteners (aspartame, acesulfame K, saccharin, sucralose, Splenda)

- Dried fruit
- Fructose
- Fruit concentrates
- Grape juice
- Honey
- Malt
- Sugar
- Sugared or commercially pickled foods containing sugar
- Sweets
- Syrups of any kind

This way of eating has several names: LCHF, banting and keto (see explanation on page 12). You may also come across the Paleo diet. This differs to LCHF in a few ways. Paleo does not allow alcohol or dairy products, apart from butter, but does allow fruit and root vegetables as well as honey. LCHF, on the other hand, restricts fruit as it is all about balancing blood sugars and reversing insulin resistance. This way of eating also only allows the approved natural sweeteners that don't raise blood sugar and are low or free from fructose, such as erythritol, xylitol and Stevia (see the Sugars and Fats chapter for more information). Dairy products are allowed on LCHF, but if you find you are not responding or losing weight, especially if you are female and premenopausal or hormonal, you may benefit from excluding dairy products (apart from butter).

At first glance, these lists may look restricting, but please believe me when I tell you that it is far from being the case. Yes, you are no longer allowed processed or junk foods, but in their place is real, honest food that not only balances your blood sugars but can also improve your health and reduce excess weight.

GET SWAPPING!

I have followed this way of eating for several years now. My diet consists of a wide range of foods, but is very traditional and family orientated. I can honestly say I don't miss much from my previous high-carb, low-fat, vegetarian lifestyle (I now eat meat). If I am honest, the only thing I really crave is crisps, which I think is the salt craving coupled with the 'crunch' that is missing from the LCHF diet. Instead, I make sure I always have some salted nuts and I love Parmesan crisps or homemade cheesy crackers. I could add pork scratchings, but I'm not a huge fan of the taste.

The following traditional meals are very easy to convert to low-carb equivalents. I hope this will help encourage you.

Traditional recipe	LCHF swap
Breakfast cereals	These are poor in nutrients and full of sugar, so swap for a healthier breakfast – (see Breakfast chapter). If you like the convenience of a cereal, opt for my LCHF granola recipe (see p69). For winter months, you can opt for a few variations to the traditional porridge. Personally, if I am in a hurry, nothing beats a bowl of full-fat yoghurt with a handful of berries and nuts
Spaghetti bolognaise	Switch spaghetti for spiralised courgettes
Curry with rice	Switch rice for broccoli or cauliflower rice
Roast dinner	Avoid potatoes, but fill up on extra veggies and meat
Pizza	There are lots of LCHF pizza recipes, including fat-head pizza, cauliflower and courgette bases
Barbecue burgers	You can make some amazing LCHF grain-free buns, or ditch the bun and have extra salad
Chilli con carne	Omit the red kidney beans. Serve with broccoli or cauliflower rice. You can also make tacos from Parmesan

Lasagne	Swap lasagne/pasta sheets for strips of courgette, aubergine, butternut squash or even bacon
Mashed potato	Cauliflower mash made with lots of cheese and butter is amazing! Use as a topping for shepherd's pie or serve with a hearty casserole
Breaded items, such as chicken nuggets, fish fingers, Scotch eggs	Make your own and use ground pork scratchings combined with Parmesan to make a crunchy coating. Simply dip into a beaten egg, then dip into the ground scratchings and bake
Bread	There are numerous recipes for LCHF breads, and I have included a few of my favourite in this book. For more recipes, search on the Internet for either keto, banting or LCHF bread recipes. Some recipes call for psyllium husk powder, which is readily available from health-food shops or online; however, some brands can turn your bread a purple colour!
Cakes and biscuits	As you will see in the bakery chapter (see p155–191), these are not forbidden, but you do have to make your own
Crisps	If you crave salty crisps, you can make your own kale crisps, or opt for salty or spicy nuts. You can also make Parmesan crisps for a cheesy salty hit (see p220)

QUICK SNACK IDEAS

This is an easy reference to quick and easy snacks you can stock up on in your fridge, ideal for when you are hungry, or to take with you to work or on a day out. Most supermarkets offer these foods, including antipasti platters, cold meats and salads. This list only includes grab-

and-go foods, but please refer to the recipes in this book for more inspiration.

- Hard-boiled eggs
- Nuts and seeds (not peanuts)
- Dark chocolate (at least 85 per cent cacao content)
- Full-fat cheese
- Pepperoni/salami/Parma ham/prosciutto
- Antipasti platters
- Biltong and beef jerky
- Salads
- Olives
- Fish, including salmon and tuna
- All meats
- Full-fat cream or natural yoghurt with berries
- Nut butters (such as almond butter) with vegetable sticks
- Parmesan crisps
- Pork scratchings

GOLDEN RULES

- Plan, plan and plan again. Planning ahead, writing shopping lists and devising meal plans really does help, especially in the first few weeks. You don't want to come home from work and have nothing to eat – that is a sure-fire way to end up eating the wrong foods.
- Don't fear the fat. We need to embrace our fat, so fill up on butter and healthy fats such as oily fish, avocado and nuts. Buy good-quality meat and eat the fat. All dairy products must be full-fat versions.
- Although this book is full of 'treat' recipes, including confectionary, cakes, biscuits and desserts, the aim is to reduce your sweet tooth naturally. These recipes are fantastic to help this become a lifestyle, but, as with everything, moderation is key. If you find you are not stabilising your blood sugar or not losing the weight you need to, it may be due to consuming too many LCHF treats.
- This diet is high fat, moderate protein and very low carbs. To reverse insulin resistance and Type 2 diabetes, you have to consume no more than 20–30g of carbohydrates per day. Note: you will find

the carbohydrate weight on the backs of most food packaging. There are also many apps to help you calculate it, such as Nutracheck and MyFitnessPal.

- Any change in diet can result in a change in bowel habits. A high-carb diet can produce very messy, sticky poos. This way of eating creates firmer, cleaner poos, but the transition may result in constipation. The best way to ensure your bowel health is in tip-top condition is to add a daily dose of bowel flora. I advise a good-quality probiotic from UK companies such as Nutrigold, NutriAdvanced, BioCare, Lamberts Healthcare or Solgar. I would strongly advise you avoid 'yoghurt' drinks, because often the healthy bacteria fails to reach the large intestine; they can also be full of sugar. A dose of vitamin C can really help get things moving, as can magnesium citrate. You must also ensure you drink enough water every day. Some of my clients find relief by taking a psyllium husk capsule daily.

- Only eat when you are hungry. We have got into the habit of snacking throughout the day, which continually stimulates an insulin response. On this way of eating, I only eat one or two meals a day, with the second meal being a light meal, and I am never hungry. As you consume more fat, you will become more satisfied, the cravings will diminish and you will stay fuller for longer.

- Change your opinion of fruit. See it as nature's candy, full of sugars, so eat it only occasionally. Berries have the least sugars, so are the best choice. Fill your plate with a good, balanced diet with plenty of vegetables, which are packed with antioxidants and phytonutrients.

- This way of eating is totally grain free. That may seem daunting at first, but it is really quite simple. Most of my clients see a dramatic difference in their health from avoiding grains, including less bloating and fewer occurrences of IBS, inflammation, skin conditions and headaches. Some fail to realise the benefits until they have a cheat meal including grains and suddenly get very poorly again.

- Don't forget salt! This way of eating can speed up the removal of electrolytes from your body as you don't retain so much water, so you need to top up with salt. We have demonised salt due to our highly processed diet. When you eat real food, you may find that you need to add salt. If you feel headachy, tired or under par, sometimes it can be an indication of too little salt or low electrolytes.

6

Store Cupboard Essentials

This is a rough guide to the ingredients you'll need when you embark on a sugar-free lifestyle. I personally try to use everyday foods, so this list is quite basic – remember you are not stocking up on lots of processed foods but making your own – even condiments.

COSTS

When you first look at this list, you may worry about the overall costs of following this way of eating. But remember, we are only consuming *real* food. You may spend more on vegetables, meat and dairy than you do on your current diet, but you won't be spending on processed foods and snacks that fill our supermarket shelves. You also won't be eating as much, as this way of eating is very satisfying. Buy in bulk where you can and use your freezer. I buy my vegetables in season and try to get what I can at local markets, so do shop around.

> 'Don't ask why healthy food is so expensive; ask why junk food is so cheap.'

FATS

This way of eating embraces natural fats and eliminates all man-made fats (see food lists in Good and Bad Foods chapter). It is really important to avoid man-made fats in order to prevent inflammation and to reverse any form of insulin resistance.

Fats to avoid

When we state to avoid all man-made fats, we are talking about processed fats, including trans fats, as well as all vegetable and seed oils (including sunflower, rapeseed, corn, sesame, canola), all margarines, vegetable shortenings and butter substitutes.

Fats to increase

We need to embrace natural fats, so include butter, coconut oil, duck fat, goose fat, lard, avocados, nuts, oily fish, cream, full-fat milk and full-fat yoghurt in your diet. These fats are in their natural state and are also stable fats. For cooking purposes, use butter, ghee, coconut oil or goose fat, as they can withstand heat, or if you prefer a liquid oil, you can opt for a good-quality olive oil or avocado oil; however, these are less stable when heated, so I would only use these as dressings. You can also use oils such as flax oil, extra-virgin olive oil or avocado oil to make your own salad dressings.

Natural sweeteners

Remember, natural sweeteners are not an excuse to eat loads and loads of sweet foods. They are a tool to help you in the transition phase to reduce your sugar cravings. Test your blood sugars after using natural sweeteners. They should not raise your blood sugar, but some people are less tolerant. The further down the road of sugar free you go, the less you will crave sweet food. You will also find you can dramatically reduce the quantity of natural sweeteners in recipes as your palate changes. See the Sugars chapters for more information on natural sweeteners.

Erythritol blend: I use Sukrin products, but you can also use the Natvia brand. You can also buy icing sugar in these ranges.

Sukrin Gold: This is an erythritol blend and a great alternative to brown sugar. I use it quite a lot to create a deeper sweet flavour. This also comes as a fibre syrup.

Xylitol: I use Total Sweet as it is available in most supermarkets, but you can buy other brands from health-food shops or online.

Stevia: I don't use stevia as I don't like the aftertaste, but there are many products available in granular or liquid forms. The best I have found is SweetLeaf liquid stevia. Always check the label to ensure it is pure stevia and not a blend of stevia and sugar.

MY STORE CUPBOARD ESSENTIALS

Nuts: I use a lot of nuts, mostly almonds, pecans, walnuts, hazelnuts, macadamia and Brazil nuts. I also use fresh nuts and blend them to make nut butters and nut flours (store nut flours in the freezer to prevent them going rancid). Nuts are also great to make your own granola and nut bars. You can also make spicy nuts as a healthy replacement to crisps.

Cake recipes often call for almond flour. This is quite expensive and at present not readily available in supermarkets in the UK. Ground almonds are much cheaper and, in my opinion, work just as well. Alternatively, you can grind your own almonds in a food processor.

Coconut: I have coconut flakes as well as desiccated coconut. I use coconut flakes in my granola and nut bars.

Coconut flour: I don't use a lot of this, preferring to use ground almonds, but it is good to have in the store cupboard and perfect if you have a nut allergy. It does absorb up to ten times its volume, so you may need to add more liquid when using this flour. Don't forget to add baking powder when making cakes.

Coconut oil: Coconut oil contains medium chain fatty acids (MCFAs), making it easy to digest and process into energy rather than being stored as fat. Many people worry about overpowering food with a coconut taste, but it honestly doesn't do this. It is not inflammatory, unlike processed oils, and is more stable when heated. Coconut oil has many health benefits, from maintaining a healthy heart right through to reducing inflammation and even preventing cancer. Buy organic cold-pressed coconut oil.

Chia seeds: These little seeds are packed with goodness. They are great to use as a thickener and they make wonderful porridge and creamy desserts.

Herbs, spices and seasonings: There are no restrictions on herbs, spices and seasonings, but do ensure any blends don't contain added sugar. I use a lot of seasonings and make my own blends. It is best if you can to buy these in bulk, as it will save money.

Cocoa/cacao: It's down to personal preference if you prefer cocoa or cacao. I prefer cacao as it is purer than cocoa, but some find it too bitter. Look for sugar-free cocoa.

Dark chocolate: You must buy the purest chocolate you can find with the least sugar. Opt for dark chocolate with a cocoa content of at least 85–95 per cent. My current favourite is 100 per cent cacao from Montezuma, Absolute Black and Chocolat Madagascar from Chococo. Hotel Chocolate also sell 100 per cent dark chocolate drops. You can also try Willies Cacao Pure Gold. Be careful when buying chocolate chips as these can contain quite a lot of sugar. Look out for the cocoa content on the packaging and, just like chocolate, aim for at least 85 per cent.

Gelatine: I use gelatine powder by Great Lakes as I like a grass-fed, natural variety. I prefer the powder, as I can also add this to biscuits and crackers to give them more crispness.

Seeds: I have a range of seeds in my cupboard: flax seeds, chia seeds, sesame seeds, pumpkin seeds and sunflower seeds are the ones I use every day. I often sauté seeds in coconut oil and add these to salads for a nice crunch and additional nutrients. I also use seeds in homemade bread and crackers, and on top of yoghurt.

Apple cider vinegar: I like to drink this every day, as it has some amazing health benefits. I also add this to bones went making bone stock as it helps to pull out the nutrients. You can use this in place of white wine vinegar in salad dressings.

Xanthan gum: This can be used as a thickener and it also helps to give a better texture to cakes and dough. It is not the easiest to use as a thickener, as it can form rather unpalatable globules, so I find it best to sprinkle in a fine mist before whisking. I tend to use arrowroot more often as a thickener.

Arrowroot: This is used in the same way you would cornflour, but it is low carb and grain free, unlike cornflour. This is available in most supermarkets.

Yeast extract: I don't like yeast extract but I use it in my cooking as it can add a good flavour. Check that your brand is sugar free.

Tinned tomatoes: You can always whip up a tasty dish if you have some tinned tomatoes. I always buy the best quality I can as I find the taste far nicer.

Tomato purée: I add this to casseroles, bolognaise, etc. I also use sun-dried tomato paste, which I make myself.

Sun-dried tomatoes in oil: I love the flavour of sun-dried tomatoes. I always have a jar to hand to add to food or make my own sun-dried tomato paste (see p250).

FRIDGE

Vegetables and salads: My fridge always has lots of salads and vegetables, including avocados – a must have! Don't let your avocados go off – you can freeze them. Frozen avocados are great to use in smoothies, guacamole and chocolate pudding.

Milk: I buy organic full-fat milk.

Cream: I buy extra-thick cream, which I use for puddings. I also have double cream to make sauces and to add to dishes. Cream is also essential for making your own ice cream.

Yoghurt: I buy full-fat natural Greek yoghurt and add berries and chopped nuts to it. Be careful as 'Greek-style' yoghurt can contain more carbohydrates than natural Greek yoghurt. I also love dairy-free coconut yoghurt, but watch the ingredients list, as some can have added sugars. I love The Coconut Collaborative and Coyo ranges.

Eggs: Absolutely vital! I probably get through a least 36 eggs a week. Eggs, especially egg yolks, are little powerhouses of nutrients and as near as we can get to a complete food. They contain omega-3 fatty acids, more so if they are free range, as well as selenium, phosphorus, vitamin A, B vitamins such as B2, B9 and B12, and carotenoids such as lutein and zeaxanthin, which can help protect us against macular degeneration and glaucoma. Eggs are great for diabetics or those with insulin resistance and obesity as they keep you full and suppress a ghrelin response (the hormone that makes you crave more food). They also contain choline, which can help reduce fatty liver and can help with some neurological conditions such as dementia, depression and cognitive behaviour.

Butter: Another essential (some people also use ghee). I do not use any margarine or spreads.

Cheese: I always have full-fat cream cheese in my fridge as I use it for puddings, pizza bases and even cakes, as it is a great binder. It is also good to use in a creamy sauce. Check out supermarket-own brands as they often contain less carbohydrates than the branded versions. I also have extra-mature Cheddar, Brie, halloumi and feta cheeses. You can also use Parmesan to make crisps or to grate onto your meals. Parmesan rinds are also worth storing in the freezer, ready to pop into a casserole, soup or frittata to increase the flavour.

Mayonnaise: I always have a jar of homemade mayonnaise in my fridge, as I love to add it to salads.

Extra-virgin olive oil: I keep this in a cool, dark cupboard as heat, light and oxygen can destroy the nutrients and turn it rancid.

Berries: For me, berries are a must-have, although I only use a small handful. I prefer raspberries and fresh blueberries. I buy frozen raspberries when they are not in season.

Lemons and limes: I cut lemons into quarters and place them in the freezer to add to drinks, as they double up as ice-cubes as well as adding a refreshing lemon flavour. I also use lemons in cakes (Lemon drizzle, Blueberry clafoutis, Lemon meringue pie – all family favourites).

Bacon: I don't eat loads of bacon, but it is always good to have in the fridge. I like to bake it until it is very crispy before chopping it into small pieces to add to a salad. I also use it in main meals and, obviously, for breakfast. I buy good-quality bacon that is not pumped with water. Try to buy from your local butcher if you can, as it won't cost much more than in the supermarkets but it will be far superior in quality.

Meat and fish: I buy free-range organic chicken. I also use beef mince, but only organic, from the supermarket or local sources recommended by my butcher. I eat steaks with salads and also like to roast a gammon joint, using the cold meat in savoury snacks and omelettes. I buy gluten-free sausages, but it's worth speaking to your butcher for grain-free options. I enjoy fresh fish, but also keep tuna steaks and salmon fillets in the freezer.

Carbonated sparkling water: This is controversial, I know, as some people believe it stops you absorbing nutrients. For me, it is a refreshing drink to have occasionally with slices of lemon and lime and can be good if you are withdrawing from fizzy drinks.

FREEZER

I try to keep a range of homemade ready meals in my freezer for when I am busy and haven't got time to put something together. Most of the recipes in this book are suitable for freezing. Always remember to label and date anything that goes in, or it can be in there for months!

Frozen berries: I tend to opt for frozen raspberries. I use these in a variety of recipes, including ice cream, desserts and even homemade berry Jelly Bears (p238).

Meat and fish: I never buy frozen meat, but I do have chicken, lardons, mince and steak in my freezer – shamefully, it is often because I don't get around to eating it in time, so I pop it in the freezer! I keep salmon fillets and tuna steaks in the freezer.

Vegetables: I have frozen peas in my freezer. I whizz up a cauliflower to make rice and pop this into small food bags and place in the freezer.

Bones: I buy a large bag of bones (about 4kg) from my butcher for around £2 a bag. This lasts me months. I slow-cook them, and then store the bone broth in the freezer in small freezer bag portions. I also place some in a silicon ice-cube tray to pop out when I need to add a touch of stock to a dish.

DRINKS

I always get asked about drinks – what is okay and what isn't. It can get a bit confusing. Ideally, you want to avoid all artificial sweeteners, especially those in fizzy drinks, as these are not only addictive, but also research now shows that reliance on these 'diet' drinks can actually lead to weight gain and can increase your appetite and craving for sweet foods. Some research even points to increased insulin resistance. Some of my clients had been drinking up to 3 litres of diet cola a day, and withdrawing from this is pretty tough!

Infused waters

I drink sparkling water with a quarter of a lemon. I cut my lemons into quarters and freeze them so that they double as ice cubes and add a lovely lemon flavour. I also like to make my own flavoured waters, adding a variety of fruit, herbs and vegetables into a water cooler or jug, which I then fill with ice and water. Great combinations include cucumber, mint and lime; slices of orange and ginger root; lemon grass, cucumber, lemon, lime and mint.

Go traditional

You can make your own lemonade following a traditional recipe, substituting the sugar with erythritol or xylitol. You can do the same for other traditional drinks, such as ginger ale.

Iced teas

You can also serve iced teas and iced coffees. Be careful with fruit teas to ensure that they have no added sugars.

Milk

Although natural, milk does contain lactose (a form of sugar). One 250ml glass of full-fat milk can contain more than 11g of carbohydrates. Low-fat milk and skimmed milk contain more than 12g of carbohydrates.

Juices and smoothies

A big no on these, unless they are predominantly vegetable based. You can make your own lower-carb smoothies using berries, avocado or natural yoghurt, but you do need to calculate the carb count, so unless you know what you are consuming, I would avoid them.

Supermarket favourites

There is a great sparking drink called Ugly (www.uglydrinks.com) available in supermarkets with no added sugar and no artificial sweeteners. It currently comes in two flavours: lemon and lime, and grapefruit and pineapple. It contains sparking water, natural flavours and citric acid – nothing else.

Alcohol

While your blood sugars are unstable, I would avoid alcohol. Once you are more settled, you can look at low-carb alcohol choices, but these should only be occasional as it will slow down your progress. Also note that those on a low-carb diet are less tolerant of alcohol, so you will feel the effects much quicker and with less alcohol.

Alcohols that contain the lowest amount of carbs are champagne and wine; beer contains the highest amount of carbs. For example, a dry white wine can contain approximately 0.5g of sugar per glass. Spirits are pretty much zero carbs, but they are dependent on what you mix them with, as mixers can really add to sugar and carb loads. I am not a fan of wine, preferring G&T or vodka. I have now converted to having a spirit, such as vodka, mixed with soda water and lime.

Caffeine

There are mixed reports on the effects of caffeine. Some state that a little is beneficial, whereas others prefer to abstain. If you suffer from a lot of stress in your life, you may have raised cortisol levels and adrenal stress, meaning too much caffeine could be detrimental. Everyone is different, so do what suits you and listen to your body.

Recipes

Breakfast

Over the last 50 years or more we have completely transformed what we eat at breakfast. What used to be a meal of eggs, kippers, bacon or kedgeree is now replaced with sugar-laden cereals, sugar-packed juice and sugary toast and jams. Is it any wonder we are all suffering from sugar overload? It is estimated that most children consume 10–15 teaspoons of sugar before they even leave for school in the morning.

- **Eggs** are an amazing complete food that not only fills you up but also provides some fantastic nutrients. It only takes minutes to rustle up a scrambled egg, and this is far more nutritious for children than sugary cereal. You can also make mini frittata muffins, which can be frozen and heated up in the morning, or made the day or evening before, or consider hard-boiled eggs. I love boiled eggs with crispy bacon soldiers. Don't forget a variety of omelettes and even fried eggs – fry them in bacon fat, butter, coconut oil or duck fat (not oils).
- **Avocados** are packed with healthy fats and are really filling. Mash avocado and serve it on low-carb, grain-free toast, or mash avocado with some hard-boiled eggs for a yummy egg–avo mayonnaise. Alternatively, serve avocado slices with bacon and egg.
- **Low-carb porridge** can be made with coconut flour, almond flour or chia seeds which, if done well, can give you a creamy porridge effect, perfect for those winter mornings when you need comfort food.
- **Pancakes** can be made with coconut flour, psyllium husk or almond flour. Serve them with berries and a dollop of yoghurt.
- **Savoury breakfast.** There is nothing in the rule book to state you must have a sweet breakfast. Bacon and eggs, smoked salmon and eggs are both great, or try my Spinach, Bacon and Egg One-Pot (see p68). The Great British fry-up is also a fantastic option as it keeps you full all day long and is an easy option when travelling.
- **Cereal.** Conventional breakfast cereals are packed with sugars and grains, so not an option for the LCHF way of eating, however, you can make your own grain-free granola, which is great with full-fat

milk or full-fat yoghurt (see page 69).

- **Breads.** Have a look at The Savoury Baker chapter for bread, bagel and muffin recipes. You can top these with low-carb, sugar-free jams (see pp242–244), chocolate spread (see p241), nut butters and curd (see p243).

SKIPPING BREAKFAST – INTERMITTENT FASTING

Some people find that they are not hungry at breakfast time, and that is perfectly fine – in fact this is the way I eat. You only eat when hungry on this way of eating (and stop when you're full). Some people find great benefit from intermittent fasting following the 16/8 schedule (fasting for 16 hours and only eating in an 8-hour time frame). For example, eat your evening meal and nothing until the following lunchtime. For more information on intermittent tasting, I recommend you look at the work of Dr Jason Fung.

Bullet-proof coffee

Some people start their day with a bullet-proof coffee. This is a combination of freshly brewed coffee whizzed in a blender along with butter and coconut oil.

SERVES 1

NUTRITIONAL INFORMATION PER SERVING
234 KCALS
24.2G FAT
0.81G NET CARBOHYDRATES
0.14G PROTEIN

180ml freshly brewed coffee
1 tbsp coconut oil or MCT oil
1 tbsp unsalted grass-fed butter

- Blend in a blender or food processor and serve immediately.

Scrambled eggs

You may think this is simple, but believe me, so many people contact me asking for a recipe. Making scrambled eggs seems to fill people with dread! The secret is a quick cook using a non-stick pan – I use a small frying pan. Do not season until just before serving. You can add cream or milk if you like (mix it in with the beaten egg), although this recipe uses just eggs.

SERVES 1 (GENEROUSLY)

NUTRITIONAL INFORMATION PER SERVING
302 KCALS
22.8G FAT
0.05G NET CARBOHYDRATES
21.6G PROTEIN

1 tsp butter or ghee
3 eggs, beaten
Salt and freshly ground black pepper

- Place a frying pan over a medium-high heat. Melt the butter gently, then add the beaten eggs.
- Use a firm spatula or wooden spoon and stir/scramble the eggs until they start to cook – this takes about 40–60 seconds. You want the eggs to be slightly underdone, as they continue to cook while on the plate. Once the eggs start to scramble and there is not too much wet egg white, they are pretty much done.
- Remove the pan from the heat and season to taste. I sometimes add some grated cheese at this point. Serve immediately.

Easy low-carb pancakes

The batter can be made in advance and kept in the fridge until breakfast. Give it a little whisk before cooking. The batter does not need any sweetener, as the sweetness comes from what you serve the pancakes with.

MAKES 6 PANCAKES

NUTRITIONAL INFORMATION PER PANCAKE
267 KCALS
21.2G FAT
3.3G NET CARBOHYDRATES
13.4G PROTEIN

6 eggs
2 tsp sugar-free vanilla extract
185g cream cheese
80g ground almonds
3 tbsp coconut flour
Zest of 1 lemon
Butter, for frying

- Put all the ingredients, except the butter, in a blender or food processor and whizz until combined. Refrigerate until ready to cook.
- Place a frying pan over a medium heat and add a knob of butter. Swirl around to ensure the butter has coated the base of the pan.
- Pour a ladleful of batter into the pan to form a pancake. Cook on both sides for 2–3 minutes until golden.
- I love these with lemon and a sprinkle of erythritol, or serve with some fresh berries and a dollop of full-fat yoghurt or cream.

Use-it-up scramble

Excuse my poor title, but it really does say it all. This is a perfect scramble to use up all those little bits and pieces lurking in your fridge. Diced ham, cooked bacon or sausage, vegetables, chilli, herbs, cheese and even leftovers from the day before. Anything goes.

SERVES 2

NUTRITIONAL INFORMATION PER SERVING
407 KCALS
29.7G FAT
2.2G NET CARBOHYDRATES
32.3G PROTEIN

2 spring onions, including green ends, diced
½ red pepper, deseeded and diced
2 tsp butter or ghee
6 eggs, beaten
3 slices of ham, diced
30g Cheddar cheese, grated (optional)
Salt and freshly ground black pepper

- Put the spring onions and red pepper in a bowl.
- Heat the butter over a medium-high heat in a non-stick pan. Add the vegetables, pour in the eggs and heat for 20 seconds. Using a spatula or wooden spoon, scramble everything together. When the eggs start to cook but are still a little moist, add the ham and cheese (if using) and combine. Season to taste.
- Remove from heat before it dries out. Serve immediately.

Avocado, bacon and egg layer

One of my absolute favourite starts to the day. I think bacon with avocado is a match made in heaven! Avocado is packed with healthy fat, keeping you fuller for longer.

SERVES 2

NUTRITIONAL INFORMATION PER SERVING
536 KCALS
43G FAT
1.3G NET CARBOHYDRATES
34.6G PROTEIN

6 rashers of back bacon
2 eggs
1 avocado, sliced
Freshly ground black pepper

- Grill or fry the bacon.
- Boil the kettle, ready for poaching the eggs. I use poach pods, because I find these quick and easy.
- Fill a saucepan with boiling water and crack an egg into each poach pod. Gently drop the pods into the water and cover the pan with a lid. Simmer for 5 minutes. (Alternatively, fill a saucepan with about 5cm boiling water and return it to the boil over a medium-high heat. Gently add the eggs to the water and simmer as before.)
- Arrange the bacon rashers on two plates. Add the avocado on top, followed by the poached eggs. Season with black pepper. Serve immediately.

Low-carb, grain-free porridge

I used to love porridge on a cold winter's morning, but this way of eating means we cannot have oats. The alternative is just as tasty, albeit a bit smoother in texture. You can opt for coconut flour or ground almonds. If you are using coconut flour, you may need to add more milk as it absorbs up to 10 times its weight. This is quite carb-heavy due to the milk, so have this occasionally only.

SERVES 2

NUTRITIONAL INFORMATION PER SERVING
264 KCALS
17.6G FAT
12.3G NET CARBOHYDRATES
10.3G PROTEIN

1 tbsp butter or ghee
300ml full-fat milk (use single cream if you want a very creamy porridge)
2 tbsp coconut flour or ground almonds
1 tbsp ground golden flaxseeds
1 tsp ground cinnamon (optional)
1 tsp erythritol or xylitol (or stevia, to taste)

- Melt the butter in a saucepan over a medium heat. Add all the remaining ingredients, retaining some of the milk/cream to adjust the thickness.
- Stir continuously until the mixture starts to thicken to your desired thickness. Serve immediately.
- You can top the porridge with a variety of toppings, including sugar-free jams (see pp242–244), berries, chopped nuts or a sprinkle of Sukrin Gold (brown erythritol granules).

Mini frittata muffins

These are so easy to make and great for a breakfast or packed lunch. You can even prep these the night before, ready to pop into the oven in the morning. I add whatever vegetables that need using up in my fridge – peppers, spring onions, courgette, tomatoes or spinach. You can also use any cooked leftover vegetables. For the purpose of the nutritional analysis, I have used 60g of spinach and 60g of red onion.

MAKES 6

NUTRITIONAL INFORMATION PER MUFFIN
126 KCALS
9.6G FAT
1.6G NET CARBOHYDRATES
8.2G PROTEIN

4 eggs, beaten
1 tbsp butter or ghee, melted, plus extra for greasing
100ml full-fat milk
1 tsp dried oregano or dried mixed herbs (optional)
Salt and freshly ground black pepper
6 tbsp finely chopped vegetables of choice
60g grated or crumbled cheese of choice

- Preheat the oven to 190°C/gas mark 5. Grease a muffin tray.
- Put the eggs in a jug with the butter, milk and herbs. Season to taste.
- Spoon the vegetables and cheese into each muffin hole, then pour over the egg mixture until they are two-thirds full.
- Bake for 20 minutes until golden. They will rise but sadly drop again once cooled. Don't worry, they still taste divine!

Spinach, bacon and egg one-pot

A really nourishing yet simple way to start the day. You can use kale or cavolo nero instead of spinach if you prefer.

SERVES 2

NUTRITIONAL INFORMATION PER SERVING
582 KCALS
44G FAT
0.41G NET CARBOHYDRATES
45G PROTEIN

1 tsp coconut oil, butter or ghee
6 rashers of bacon
60g baby leaf spinach
4 eggs
50g feta cheese, crumbled
Salt and freshly ground black pepper

- Heat the coconut oil in a frying pan over a medium heat. Add the bacon, making sure it covers the base of the pan. Fry gently on both sides for a few minutes.
- Add the spinach on top of the bacon. Crack the eggs onto the spinach and top with the feta. Season to taste.
- Cover the pan with a lid and cook for 5–8 minutes until the eggs are cooked. Serve immediately.

Choco-nutty granola

This granola is really easy to make, and there is nothing stopping you doubling or tripling the quantities to make up a large batch as it keeps well in a sealed, airtight container.

MAKES 15 SERVINGS

NUTRITIONAL INFORMATION PER 55G SERVING
347 KCALS
32G FAT
4G NET CARBOHYDRATES
8.2G PROTEIN

300g mixed nuts (brazils, hazelnuts, almonds, macadamia, walnuts)
100g pecan nuts (these add a sweetness kids love)
75g flaked almonds
100g unsweetened coconut flakes
75g sunflower seeds
75g pumpkin seeds
40g coconut oil, melted
2 tbsp unsweetened cocoa or cacao powder
2 tbsp xylitol or erythritol (or to taste)

- Preheat the oven to 150°C/gas mark 2.
- Put the mixed nuts in a freezer bag and bash with a rolling pin into small bite-size pieces. I like doing this as it takes out my frustrations! Don't use a food processor as it will over-process the nuts and if you are not careful you will end up with nutty dust!
- Put the crushed nuts into a bowl and add the other nuts, coconut flakes and seeds.
- Pour the melted coconut oil into a jug, then add the cocoa and sweetener and combine well. Pour this over the nut and seed mix and stir well until the oil coats all the nuts.
- Tip the nut mixture onto a large baking tray (you may need two trays) and spread evenly to cover the tray.
- Bake for 5 minutes before turning the nuts, then bake for a further 5 minutes.
- Remove from the oven and cool before storing in an airtight container.

Basic chia porridge

You have probably seen chia seeds featured in the press. These little seeds are packed full of protein. They absorb liquid, so are a great thickener, which is why I use them in my sugar-free jams. This recipe is for a basic chai porridge – you can add more flavours, such as fruit, a spoonful of cacao or cocoa, or flaked coconut. Top with whatever takes your fancy.

This needs to be prepared at least 1 hour in advance, but ideally the night before.

SERVES 2

NUTRITIONAL INFORMATION PER SERVING
219 KCALS
13.9G FAT
7.8G NET CARBOHYDRATES
9.6G PROTEIN

250ml full-fat milk (use coconut or almond milk if you prefer)
60g chia seeds
1 tsp sugar-free vanilla extract (optional)
Sprinkle of sweetener, to taste (I use Sukrin Gold)

- Put the milk and chia seeds in a bowl or jug. Stir in the vanilla (if using). Leave to rest in the fridge for 1 hour or overnight.
- You can eat this porridge hot or cold. I prefer it hot, so I gently warm it in a saucepan until heated through, adding more milk if necessary.
- Finish with a sprinkle of sweetener. If you like, top with some nuts and berries.

Cinnamon nut granola

This cinnamon nut granola is one of my favourites. It is delicious as a breakfast or as a topping for a fruit crumble, but I like it best when served with a dollop of thick natural Greek yoghurt with some blueberries. As with all the granolas, store in an airtight container.

MAKES ABOUT 15 SERVINGS

NUTRITIONAL INFORMATION PER 55G SERVING
360 KCALS
33.3G FAT
3.7G NET CARBOHYDRATES
8.6G PROTEIN

300g mixed nuts (brazils, hazelnuts, almonds, macadamia, walnuts)
100g pecan nuts
60g flaked almonds
100g coconut flakes
75g sunflower seeds
75g pumpkin seeds
50g flaxseeds
40g coconut oil, melted
2 tsp ground cinnamon
1/2 tsp ground mixed spice
1/2 tsp allspice
2 tbsp xylitol or erythritol (or to taste)

- Preheat the oven to 150°C/gas mark 2.
- Put the mixed nuts in a freezer bag and bash with a rolling pin into small bite-size pieces.
- Put the crushed nuts into a bowl and add the other nuts, coconut flakes and seeds.
- Pour the melted coconut oil in a jug, then add the cinnamon, spices and sweetener, and combine well. Pour this over the nut and seed mix, and stir well until the oil coats all the nuts.
- Tip the nut mixture onto a large baking tray (you may need two trays) and spread evenly to cover the tray.
- Bake for 5 minutes before turning the nuts, then bake for a further 5 minutes.
- Remove from the oven and cool before storing in an airtight container.

Sweet berry frittata

I've popped this into the breakfast chapter, but if I am honest, I also enjoy this for a quick supper if I don't have much of an appetite. I love it served with cream or Greek yoghurt. I don't bother with sweetener, but if you are new to sugar free, you may want to add some xylitol, erythritol or a touch of stevia.

SERVES 2

NUTRITIONAL INFORMATION PER SERVING
272 KCALS
22.1G FAT
3.1G NET CARBOHYDRATES
13.7G PROTEIN

3 eggs, beaten
150ml single cream or full-fat milk
1 tsp xylitol or erythritol (optional)
Butter or coconut oil, for frying
Handful of berries (raspberry and blueberries are best)

- Preheat the grill.
- Beat the eggs, cream and sweetener (if using) together in a jug.
- Melt a little butter in a frying pan over a medium heat. Pour the egg mixture into the pan and tip the pan from side to side to spread the mixture. Cook for 1–2 minutes until starting to set before dropping in the berries. Cook for a further minute, then remove from the heat.
- Pop under the grill for 5 minutes, or until puffed up and golden. Serve hot or cold with Greek yoghurt or double cream.

Lunch Ideas

So, what is the best thing to have for lunch? It is quite simple: **Eat Real Food.** We have lost the skills to make food from scratch and become more and more reliant on quick meal fixes that are, due to the manufacturing processes, often devoid of nutrients and full of sugar.

IDEAS FOR PACKED LUNCHES

Packed lunches can be mind-numbingly dull and monotonous. We can make them healthy and tasty, but it takes more time and effort, which we may not always have. Rushing to fill your lunchbox with 5 minutes to spare before you dash out the front door is not a good way to create a healthy, sugar-free lunch. The secret, as always, is to plan ahead.

Remember the foods that are healthy on your sugar-free, low-carb journey and use these to bulk out your packed lunch:

- **Eggs:** These can be hard boiled, mixed with mayo to make egg mayonnaise, low-carb Scotch eggs or mini frittatas and quiches.
- **Nuts:** These are far healthier than crisps. See the savoury snacks chapter for healthy crisps and flavoured nut recipes. Some schools have a no-nut policy, so check before you add these to your children's lunches.
- **Cheese:** You can buy individually wrapped cheese, which is very filling and perfect for a quick snack.
- **Veg sticks:** These are great to munch on, especially with a little pot of dip.
- **Meats:** If using up your meat leftovers, roast chicken makes a great sandwich or Caesar salad. I have also made the Chicken Fajitas (see p124) and the Chicken Schnitzel (see p107) in this book and eaten them cold with a salad. Kids really love these. I bake bacon in the oven (I find it is crispier doing it this way) and then store it in the fridge. It's great in sandwiches or chopped and added to salads. Kids love cold mini sausages, but check the ingredients as they can contain lots of sugars and grains.

- **Tuna:** A bit smelly, but tuna is very nutritious. I make up tuna mayonnaise and store it in little pots to have with a salad.
- **Low-carb, grain-free bread:** There are lots of low-carb bread recipes on the internet and these vary in success. I have had many a purple loaf due to psyllium husk issues! I prefer my Grain-free Low-carb Crackers (see p162) – great with dips and toppings.
- **Pizza:** Check out the recipes in the Healthier Fast Food chapter as these are great cold in packed lunches.
- **Salads:** Fill your lunchbox with salad, but don't add the salad dressing until you are just about to eat or you will end up with a soggy mess by lunchtime.
- **Leftovers:** If you have access to a kitchen at work, why not take in your own food? Spend a day batch-cooking, divide into individual portions and pop into the freezer. Get into the habit of making slightly more when you cook your meals, and pop the leftovers into the freezer ready for another meal or lunch.
- **Treats:** See the bakery chapters (pages 155–190) for more ideas.
- **Yoghurts:** Buy full-fat natural Greek yoghurt. Add your own fruit, nuts or seeds to suit.

It's a wrap!

These are as near as you can get to low-carb, grain-free tortilla wraps. They are softer than shop-bought ones, but still lovely with spicy chicken or stuffed with your favourite filling. Ensure you use a good-quality frying pan to make these – it really does make life easier when they slide off without sticking!

MAKES 4

NUTRITIONAL INFORMATION PER WRAP
345 KCALS
27G FAT
3.7G NET CARBOHYDRATES
22G PROTEIN

3 tbsp double cream
2 tbsp cold water
2 eggs, beaten
3 egg whites
4 tbsp coconut flour
50g finely grated mozzarella cheese
½ tsp paprika
½ tsp oregano
Salt and freshly ground black pepper
Coconut oil or butter, for frying

- Mix all the ingredients, except the oil, together in a bowl using a balloon whisk.
- Heat a little coconut oil in a frying pan and ensure the base is evenly and lightly coated.
- Spoon a ladleful of batter into the pan, tilting the pan at various angles until it is evenly covered. You want a thin layer all over the base of the pan, a little thicker than an English pancake or French crêpe. Cook for 3–5 minutes until golden on both sides.
- Place on a piece of kitchen paper and repeat with the remaining batter. You can store the wraps in the fridge up to 3 days, ensuring they are separated by a sheet of baking parchment. Alternatively, serve warm with your favourite filling.

Broccoli and Stilton soup

Broccoli and Stilton soup is delicious and perfect for low carbers, as it is low in carbohydrates and high in healthy fat, keeping you full for hours. This recipe also freezes well, so why not double up the recipe and store some extra portions in the freezer.

SERVES 6

NUTRITIONAL INFORMATION PER SERVING
307 KCALS
17.4G FAT
8.4G NET CARBOHYDRATES
19.3G PROTEIN

1 tsp coconut oil or butter or ghee
1 red onion, finely chopped
1 stick of celery, finely chopped
450ml hot vegetable, chicken or bone stock
700g broccoli (about 2 heads), roughly chopped
150g Stilton or blue cheese
Salt and freshly ground black pepper

- Put the coconut oil in a saucepan. Add the onion and celery, and cook until they start to soften.
- Add the stock and broccoli, and cook for 10 minutes until the broccoli is cooked.
- Add the Stilton and stir well until dissolved. Use a stick blender to blend until smooth, and season to taste before serving.

Chicken, cumin and harissa soup

This is a lovely soup, perfect as a winter warmer. You can buy harissa paste or seasoning, but ensure it is free from sugar. This soup isn't blended, so make sure you chop everything evenly.

SERVES 5

NUTRITIONAL INFORMATION PER SERVING
152 KCALS
2.8G FAT
6.5G NET CARBOHYDRATES
24.3G PROTEIN

2 tsp butter or coconut oil
1 red onion, finely chopped
2 cloves of garlic, finely chopped
1 red pepper, deseeded and finely chopped
400g chicken fillets, cut into small chunks
1 tsp ground cumin
1 tsp paprika
2 tsp harissa paste
400g tin chopped tomatoes
500ml hot bone or chicken stock
Small handful of chopped coriander, plus extra to garnish

- Heat the butter in a saucepan over a medium heat and cook the onion, garlic and red pepper until they start to soften.
- Add the chicken and cook until it turns white before adding the remaining ingredients. Simmer for 20 minutes.
- To serve, ladle into bowls and garnish with coriander.

Mediterranean-style tortilla

This is an ideal dish for using up any leftover vegetables – anything goes, so experiment!

SERVES 4

NUTRITIONAL INFORMATION PER SERVING
345 KCALS
27G FAT
3.7G NET CARBOHYDRATES
22G PROTEIN

5 eggs
1 bunch of spring onions, finely chopped
1 red pepper, deseeded and diced or thinly sliced
150g pancetta, diced
4 sun-dried tomatoes, chopped
50g Parmesan cheese, grated
Small handful of fresh herbs (basil, oregano or thyme are good)
Salt and freshly ground black pepper

- Preheat the oven to 200°C/gas mark 6. Line a 20cm round ovenproof dish with baking parchment.
- Add the eggs to a large bowl and beat well. Add the remaining ingredients and combine.
- Pour the mixture into the prepared dish and bake for 20–25 minutes until firm. Serve hot or cold with salad.

Crustless spinach and feta pie

Serve this with a selection of fresh salad dishes – the perfect dish for a warm summer's evening.

SERVES 6

NUTRITIONAL INFORMATION PER SERVING
222 KCALS
18.6G FAT
1G NET CARBOHYDRATE
12.2G PROTEIN

400g baby leaf spinach, roughly torn
300g feta cheese, crumbled
2 eggs, beaten
Finely grated nutmeg, to taste
50g grated mature Cheddar (optional)
Sesame seeds, for sprinkling
Freshly ground black pepper

- Preheat the oven to 200°C/gas mark 6. Grease a 20cm pie dish.
- Put the spinach in a colander and rinse it with just-boiled water until the spinach starts to wilt, then gently squeeze out the water. Put it in a mixing bowl. Add the feta, beaten eggs and nutmeg. If you like a cheesy dish, you can also add 50g of grated mature Cheddar. Season well with black pepper. Transfer to the prepared pie dish. Finish with a sprinkle of sesame seeds.
- Bake for 25–30 minutes until golden and crisp. Serve hot or cold.

Cauliflower cheese and bacon soup

This soup is very comforting and filling – perfect when you are feeling in need of a food 'hug'. You can top the soup with crispy bacon bits. Delicious!

SERVES 6

NUTRITIONAL INFORMATION PER SERVING
369 KCALS
31.5G FAT
6.9G NET CARBOHYDRATES
13G PROTEIN

2 tsp butter or ghee
1 onion, finely chopped
100g smoked bacon lardons
1 stick of celery, finely chopped
350ml hot vegetable, chicken or bone stock
600g cauliflower, roughly chopped
200ml double cream
125g mature Cheddar cheese, grated
Freshly ground black pepper

- Melt the butter in a saucepan over a medium heat. Add the onion, lardons and celery, and cook until they start to soften.
- Add the stock and cauliflower, and cook for 15 minutes until the cauliflower is cooked.
- Add the cream and cheese, and stir well until dissolved. Use a stick blender to blend until smooth. Season with black pepper before serving.

Green squeak patties

Here is a great way to get some extra veg into your diet and to use up any leftovers you may have in your fridge. You can use cauliflower, broccoli, greens or even courgettes for these little beauties. I prefer cauliflower or broccoli, but that is personal choice. I like to cook them until golden and crispy.

MAKES 10

NUTRITIONAL INFORMATION PER PATTY
104 KCALS
7.6G FAT
1.2G NET CARBOHYDRATES
7.4G PROTEIN

1 head of cauliflower or broccoli (approx. 300g)
6 slices of bacon or pancetta, finely chopped
Butter or coconut oil, for frying
½ bunch of spring onions, finely chopped
100g mature Cheddar cheese, grated
1 egg, beaten
1 teaspoon wholegrain mustard
Salt and freshly ground black pepper

- Steam the cauliflower or broccoli until soft. Meanwhile, fry the bacon in a little butter until nice and crispy.
- Put the cauliflower or broccoli in a bowl and mash (or use a food processor). Add the spring onions, cheese, cooked bacon, egg and mustard to the bowl and mash/combine together thoroughly. Season to taste.
- Form the mixture into 10 patties – don't worry if they are lumpy, as this is part of their charm.
- Bake or fry the patties on both sides until golden. I bake them for 20 minutes at 180°C/gas mark 4.

Celery and Stilton soup

I love this soup, as it has a nice creamy texture and is not too cheesy. My son loves it too, although I have to keep the Stilton a secret – if he saw me put it in, he wouldn't eat it! The blue cheese is quite salty, so you don't need to add extra salt.

SERVES 4

NUTRITIONAL INFORMATION PER SERVING
338 KCALS
31.5G FAT
5.1G NET CARBOHYDRATES
7.4G PROTEIN

25g butter or coconut oil
1 onion, finely chopped
450g celery, finely diced
500ml hot bone or vegetable stock
150g Stilton cheese, crumbled
200ml double cream
Salt and freshly ground black pepper

- Heat the butter in a saucepan and fry the onion for 2 minutes. Add the celery and stock and simmer over a low heat for 15 minutes.
- Add the Stilton and double cream, and stir until melted and combined. Blend using a stick blender and season to taste. Serve immediately or set aside until ready to eat.
- This soup freezes well. Alternatively, it can be refrigerated in an airtight container for two to three days.

Crustless egg and bacon quiche

I remember my mum making this quiche for Sunday tea. It was always a favourite of mine, along with cheese and onion quiche. You can use pancetta if you prefer.

CUTS INTO 8 SLICES

NUTRITIONAL INFORMATION PER SLICE
300 KCALS
26.7G FAT
0.66G NET CARBOHYDRATES
14G PROTEIN

4 rashers of smoked bacon, cooked and diced
1 bunch of spring onions, finely chopped
120g mature Cheddar cheese, grated
6 eggs, beaten
200ml double cream
1 tsp dried oregano
1 tsp fresh parsley, chopped
Salt and freshly ground black pepper

- Preheat the oven to 190°C/gas mark 5.
- Put the bacon pieces in a 20cm ovenproof dish. Top with the spring onions and cheese.
- Mix the eggs and cream together in a jug until combined. Add the herbs and season to taste. Pour into the dish.
- Bake for 30–40 minutes until the quiche has risen and is golden on top. Eat hot or cold.

Low-carb, grain-free Scotch eggs

I love these, and they are so worth the time it takes to make them. Be careful when choosing your sausage meat as most contain sugars and grains. Speak to your butcher to get the best quality, as it will make a huge difference.

MAKES 4

NUTRITIONAL INFORMATION PER SCOTCH EGG
711 KCALS
55G FAT
2.7G NET CARBOHYDRATES
52G PROTEIN

5 eggs
400g good-quality sausage meat
1 tsp dried thyme
1 tsp dried parsley
1 tsp dried sage
200g pork scratchings, crushed
2 tsp paprika
50g Parmesan cheese, grated (optional)
Olive oil, for frying
Salt and freshly ground black pepper

- Boil the kettle. Put 4 of the eggs in a saucepan. Pour over the boiling water and place over a medium heat. Boil for 6 minutes. Remove from the heat, drain and run the eggs under cold running water. Leave them in the saucepan filled with cold water.
- While the eggs are cooling, put the sausage meat in a bowl. Add the thyme, parsley and sage, and season to taste.
- Peel the eggs, discarding the shells.
- Divide the sausage meat into four equal portions and form each piece into a ball. Flatten each ball as much as you can. Put the egg in the centre and wrap the sausage meat around the egg firmly until it is completely covered.
- Beat the remaining egg in a bowl. Put the pork scratchings, paprika and Parmesan in a separate bowl, season with pepper and combine.
- This is where it can get messy! Dip each Scotch egg into the egg mixture before coating it in the pork scratchings. Place on a sheet of greaseproof paper until you are ready to fry.
- Heat 5–6cm of oil in a saucepan or use a deep-fat fryer at a medium-high heat. Add the Scotch eggs, turning until the eggs are golden and crispy.
- Remove from the pan using a slotted spoon and place on kitchen paper to drain. When cool, store in an airtight container for up to five days in the fridge.

Feel-good chicken and vegetable soup

This is a great soup to pick you up when you are feeling under par. I add more chilli and grated ginger when I am suffering from a cold or flu – it works a treat. There are quite a few vegetables in this soup, but really, it is the perfect soup to use up any vegetables you may have in your fridge, so feel free to adapt the recipe. This soup is particularly suitable to make in a slow cooker.

SERVES 6

NUTRITIONAL INFORMATION PER SERVING
201 KCALS
10.5G FAT
6.8G NET CARBOHYDRATES
18.1G PROTEIN

1 tsp coconut oil
1 red onion, finely chopped
2 cloves of garlic, chopped
1 chilli, diced
2cm piece of ginger, peeled and finely chopped (optional)
100g diced lardons or pancetta
250g chicken fillet, diced
1 stick of celery, diced
1 red pepper, deseeded and diced
50g green beans, diced
1 courgette, diced
400g tin chopped tomatoes
2 tsp paprika
1 tsp thyme
750ml hot chicken or bone stock
Salt and freshly ground black pepper

- Preheat the slow cooker following the manufacturer's instructions.
- I have a multi-cooker, which has a sauté facility – perfect for this soup – but if you don't have one, you will need to sauté the first few ingredients in a pan: in a saucepan, heat the coconut oil and fry the onion, garlic, chilli, ginger, lardons and chicken until sealed.
- Put all the remaining ingredients into the slow cooker and turn on to high. Cook for 6 hours. If cooking in a saucepan, simmer for 25 minutes. If you like, serve topped with grated cheese.

Main Meals

We are following a low-carb, grain-free, sugar-free way of eating. We also need to try to limit root vegetables due to their high starch content. But don't worry – this chapter has all your family favourites and should give you the confidence to adapt any of your own recipes. Enjoy lasagne, spag bol, fish fingers, cottage pie and chilli con carne, all made with a low-carb twist, but all just as delicious.

Low-carb lasagne

You don't need pasta sheets to make a low-carb lasagne; in fact, there is a variety of options to choose from. This recipe opts for aubergine slices, but you can use courgette, butternut squash, or even cooked bacon rashers. You can also make this in advance and freeze it until you are ready to cook – ensure it is thoroughly defrosted before placing it in the oven.

SERVES 6

NUTRITIONAL INFORMATION PER SERVING
919 KCALS
85G FAT
9.5G NET CARBOHYDRATES
26.9G PROTEIN

2 aubergines
1 tsp coconut oil
1 red onion, finely chopped
2–3 cloves of garlic, to taste, finely chopped
1 red pepper, finely chopped
100g lardons or pancetta
400g beef mince
200ml beef bone stock
400g tin chopped tomatoes
2 tsp tomato purée
2 tsp dried oregano
2 tsp paprika
250ml double cream
250ml mascarpone cheese
100g mature Cheddar cheese, grated
25g Parmesan cheese, grated
Salt and freshly ground black pepper

- Slice the aubergines and put them on a plate or tray. Sprinkle with salt and set aside.
- Heat the coconut oil in a frying pan and fry the onion until soft and translucent. Add the garlic and red pepper, and cook for a further 2 minutes.
- Add the lardons and beef mince, and cook until browned. Add the stock and cook for 2 more minutes.
- Stir in the tomatoes and tomato purée. Add the oregano and paprika, and season with black pepper. Simmer for 10 minutes.
- Preheat the oven to 180°C/gas mark 4.
- Shake off the salt and pat the aubergines dry with kitchen paper.
- Mix the cream, mascarpone and Cheddar together in a bowl. Season.
- Spread a little of the bolognaise mixture in the base of a 20cm square ovenproof dish. Add a layer of aubergine, then a thin layer of the cream mixture. Repeat the layers, finishing with the cream mixture. Sprinkle with the Parmesan.
- Bake for 30 minutes until bubbling. Serve with a green salad.

Ham and leek cheesy bake

This is a really comforting supper, and one of my favourites. The rich, cheesy sauce also goes well with broccoli and cauliflower. This dish can be frozen.

SERVES 4

NUTRITIONAL INFORMATION PER SERVING
746 KCALS
69G FAT
5.5G NET CARBOHYDRATES
23G PROTEIN

4 leeks, trimmed top and tail

For the cheese sauce
400ml double cream
75g mature Cheddar cheese, grated
½ tsp mustard powder
1 tsp arrowroot powder (optional)
4 slices of thick, good-quality ham or bacon
40g Parmesan cheese, grated
Freshly ground black pepper

- Preheat the oven to 200°C/gas mark 6.
- Cut the leeks to 10–12.5cm in length and steam for 5–8 minutes until just tender.
- Meanwhile, make the sauce. Heat the cream in a saucepan and stir in the cheese and mustard powder.
- Season with black pepper. If you need to thicken the sauce, put 1 teaspoon of arrowroot mixed with a little water in a cup. Stir well before adding this to the cream, stirring well until it thickens.
- Remove the leeks from the steamer and wrap 1–2 slices of ham or bacon around each leek. Lay them in the base of a 20cm square ovenproof dish.
- Pour the cheese sauce over the leeks and top with the Parmesan.
- Bake for 20 minutes until golden and bubbling.

Creamy bacon and thyme chicken

This is one of my family's favourite dishes and is very easy to make – my husband says he virtually inhales it, he eats it so fast! I serve this with steamed green vegetables. It is very filling.

SERVES 4

NUTRITIONAL INFORMATION PER SERVING
689 KCALS
59G FAT
6.7G NET CARBOHYDRATES
27.7G PROTEIN

1 tsp coconut oil, olive oil or butter
2 cloves of garlic, crushed
1 red onion, finely diced
1 leek, finely chopped
150g smoked pancetta, diced
4 chicken breasts, halved
150ml white wine (optional)
2 tsp chicken seasoning
2 sprigs of thyme
2 tsp dried oregano
1 tsp dried or 1 tbsp chopped fresh parsley
300ml double cream
Salt and freshly ground black pepper

- Heat the oil in a frying pan over a medium heat. Add the garlic, onion, leeks and pancetta, and cook for 5 minutes.
- Add the chicken breasts and cook for 8–10 minutes until the outside of the chicken is white on all sides.
- Add the wine (if using), chicken seasoning and herbs. Season to taste. Cover with a lid, reduce the heat to low and cook for 10 minutes.
- Remove the lid and stir in the cream. Cook over a low heat for a further 15–20 minutes until the chicken is cooked through.
- Serve with steamed seasonal green vegetables.

Spicy chicken balls

I used to love falafels, but this way of eating does not allow pulses, so I created this recipe. I love this served with salad for a quick lunch, but it can also be served as a side dish with a curry.

SERVES 6

NUTRITIONAL INFORMATION PER SERVING
142 KCALS
4.1G FAT
1.7G NET CARBOHYDRATES
21.5G PROTEIN

400g chicken mince
1 small onion, finely chopped
2 cloves of garlic, crushed
1 fresh chilli, finely chopped
½ tsp dried mint
½–1 tsp chilli powder, to taste
½ tsp ground cumin
1 tsp ground coriander
1 heaped tbsp almond butter
Butter or coconut oil, for frying
Seasoning, to taste

- Put all the ingredients, except the butter, in a bowl and combine well.
- Use your hands to form the mixture into 12 even-sized balls and place on a plate. Refrigerate until you are ready to cook.
- Heat a little butter in a frying pan. Add the chicken balls and cook until golden brown all over.
- Place on kitchen paper to drain and serve with a salad or as a side dish with a curry.

Vegetarian nut roast

This is a fantastic recipe for a roast or Christmas dinner. It has always been popular with both meat eaters and vegetarians. Using a food processor really speeds up the preparation process.

SERVES 6
VEGETARIAN

NUTRITIONAL INFORMATION PER SERVING
293 KCALS
25.1G FAT
3.6G NET CARBOHYDRATES
10.4G PROTEIN

10g butter or ghee
1 red onion, finely chopped
2 cloves of garlic, crushed
200g Brazil nuts, chopped (a processor makes this job easier)
250g chestnut mushrooms, chopped
2 tsp yeast extract
1 tsp dried oregano
25g ground almonds or coconut flour
Salt and freshly ground black pepper

- Preheat the oven to 190°C/gas mark 5. Line a 1lb loaf tin with baking parchment.
- Heat the butter in a frying pan and fry the onion and garlic until translucent.
- Add the nuts and mushrooms, and cook for 5 minutes.
- Add the yeast extract and oregano, followed by the ground almonds. Season to taste.
- Tip the mixture into the prepared loaf tin and press down to form a firm base. Bake for 40 minutes or until golden on top.

Top tip: This nut roast can be prepared in advance and frozen (before baking).

Baked stuffed aubergines

This is a great vegetarian dish that can be prepared in advance. If you prefer a meat dish, you can stuff the aubergine halves with bolognaise (p96) or chilli (p104) and sprinkle with grated cheese before baking.

SERVES 4
VEGETARIAN

NUTRITIONAL INFORMATION PER SERVING
229 KCALS
16G FAT
8.1G NET CARBOHYDRATES
10.4G PROTEIN

2 aubergines
Olive oil, for brushing
20g butter or ghee
1 red onion, diced
1 red pepper, deseeded and diced
2 cloves of garlic, diced
10 cherry tomatoes, halved
2 tbsp sun-dried tomato paste (sugar free)
1 tsp paprika
1 tsp dried oregano
80g baby leaf spinach
125g mozzarella cheese, diced
50g Parmesan cheese, grated
Salt and freshly ground black pepper

- Preheat the oven to 180°C/gas mark 4.
- Cut the aubergines in half lengthways. Scoop out, dice and reserve the flesh.
- Brush the aubergine shells with a little olive oil. Season to taste. Place on a baking tray and cover with foil. Bake for 10 minutes.
- Meanwhile, heat the butter in a frying pan. Add the onion, red pepper and garlic, and cook over a medium heat until everything starts to soften.
- Add the aubergine flesh, cherry tomatoes, sun-dried tomato paste, paprika and oregano. Season to taste.
- Cook for 5–10 minutes until softened. Don't forget to remove the aubergines from the oven!
- Remove the frying pan from the heat and stir in the spinach and mozzarella.
- Stuff the aubergines and sprinkle with the Parmesan.
- Return to the oven and bake for 15 minutes or until golden. Serve with a green salad.

Courgetti bolognaise

I think it is important to keep to traditional family favourites, especially when dieting. Food is not just about taste; it is also about satisfying the mind.

SERVES 6

NUTRITIONAL INFORMATION PER SERVING
301 KCALS
18.6G FAT
10.3G NET CARBOHYDRATES
20G PROTEIN

1 tsp coconut oil
1 red onion, finely chopped
2–3 cloves of garlic, to taste, finely chopped
1 red pepper, deseeded and finely chopped
100g lardons or pancetta
400g beef mince
200ml beef bone stock (or red wine)
400g tin chopped tomatoes
2 tsp tomato paste
75g chestnut or button mushrooms, chopped
2 tsp dried oregano
Freshly ground black pepper

- Heat the oil in a frying pan over a medium heat and fry the onion until soft and translucent.
- Add the garlic and red pepper, and cook for a further 2 minutes.
- Add the lardons and beef mince, and cook until browned. Add the stock (or wine) and cook for a further 2 minutes.
- Stir in the tomatoes and tomato paste. Add the mushrooms and oregano, and season with black pepper. Simmer very gently for 15 minutes. Serve on a bed of courgette spaghetti, which you can make using a hand-held spiraliser.

Beef and mushroom stroganoff

I featured this recipe in one of my other books and a reviewer said that it was better than Jamie Oliver's – praise indeed. I will leave you to decide on that one!

SERVES 4

NUTRITIONAL INFORMATION PER SERVING
508 KCALS
35G FAT
6.5G NET CARBOHYDRATES
31G PROTEIN

Coconut oil, or butter or ghee
1 large red onion, finely chopped
2–3 cloves of garlic, to taste, crushed
500g beef steak (ideally rump), cut into chunks
300g chestnut mushrooms, sliced
2 tsp paprika
2 tsp Dijon mustard
200ml white wine
2 tsp chopped fresh tarragon
200ml double cream

- Heat the oil in a large frying pan over a medium heat and cook the onion and garlic for 1 minute. Add the beef and cook for 3–4 minutes, ensuring it is browned all over.
- Add the mushrooms, paprika and mustard. Stir well, add the wine and cook for a further 2 minutes.
- Add the tarragon and cook for 2–3 minutes more.
- Just before serving, stir in the cream to form a creamy sauce, heating through until bubbling. Serve on a bed of cauliflower rice (p146).

Salmon fish cakes

These are really simple but tasty fish cakes. You can use tinned salmon if you prefer, although fresh is far tastier. Omega-rich oily fish decreases the production of inflammatory proteins, so these cakes have great anti-inflammatory properties.

SERVES 4

NUTRITIONAL INFORMATION PER SERVING
248 KCALS
16.5G FAT
1.2G NET CARBOHYDRATE
22.9G PROTEIN

400g salmon fillets
Juice of ½ lemon, plus extra to season
Freshly ground black pepper
¼–⅓ head of cauliflower or broccoli for 4 tbsp cauliflower or
  broccoli mash (p148)
3 spring onions, very finely chopped
2 tsp each of chopped fresh dill and tarragon
1 egg, beaten, if needed
Olive oil, for brushing

- Season the salmon fillets with some lemon juice and black pepper. Pop under the grill and cook for 5–6 minutes. You will know when the salmon is cooked as it will flake when touched with a fork.
- Combine the salmon, cauliflower mash, spring onions, lemon juice and herbs together in a bowl. Season to taste. Add a little beaten egg to bind the mixture, if needed.
- Form the mixture into four cakes. Place on baking parchment and refrigerate for 10 minutes, or until needed.
- Remove the cakes from the fridge, brush with a light coating of oil and grill both sides until browned. Or you can spray a frying pan with coconut or olive oil, and fry gently until browned on both sides. Serve with a green salad.

Stuffed pork tenderloin

A great family roast. Serve with steamed vegetables and homemade gravy.

SERVES 6

NUTRITIONAL INFORMATION PER SERVING
555 KCALS
47G FAT
5.2G NET CARBOHYDRATES
28G PROTEIN

75g pork scratchings, crushed
1 red onion, finely chopped
2–3 cloves of garlic, to taste, finely chopped
150g lardons or pancetta
50g pine nuts
80g spinach leaves
6 sun-dried tomatoes (in oil), chopped
Handful of fresh herbs (sage, thyme, oregano or parsley), chopped
700g pork tenderloin, butterflied and pounded flat
1 tbsp olive oil
Sea salt and freshly ground black pepper

- Preheat the oven to 200°C/gas mark 6.
- In a mixing bowl, add the pork scratchings, onion, garlic, lardons, pine nuts, spinach, sun-dried tomatoes and herbs. Combine well and season to taste.
- Place the stuffing on the meat and roll tightly. Use water-soaked string to tie the loin securely.
- Rub the skin with the oil and sprinkle with sea salt and black pepper.
- Place the loin on a baking or roasting tray and roast for 20 minutes. Reduce the temperature to 180°C/gas mark 4 and cook for 45 minutes. If the meat starts to darken too much while cooking, cover it tightly with foil.
- Use a meat thermometer to check if the meat is cooked (the reading should be around 65°C), or check the juices – if they run clear, it should be cooked.
- Remove from the oven and cover loosely with foil. Leave to rest for 10–15 minutes before carving.

Stuffed mushroom, bacon and goat's cheese salad

I love this combination. You can prepare this dish in advance and keep it in the fridge until you are ready to grill or oven bake. Opt for peppery salad leaves such as spinach, rocket and watercress as these complement the dish well.

SERVES 4

NUTRITIONAL INFORMATION PER SERVING
657 KCALS
57G FAT
7.6G NET CARBOHYDRATES
19.8G PROTEIN

4 large portobello mushrooms, stalks removed
Coconut oil, melted, or avocado oil, for brushing
3 tbsp cream cheese
40g baby leaf spinach, wilted and chopped
110g goat's cheese, crumbled
100g mixed leaf salad, washed
6 rashers of bacon, cooked until very crispy, then diced
1 red onion, thinly sliced
1 avocado, diced

For the dressing
100ml extra-virgin olive oil, flax oil or avocado oil
3 tbsp white wine vinegar
2 tbsp finely chopped chives
Salt and freshly ground black pepper

- Preheat the oven to 190°C/gas mark 5.
- Place the mushrooms on a baking tray and brush with a little oil. Bake for 5 minutes to soften.
- Put the spinach in a colander and rinse it with just-boiled water until the spinach starts to wilt, then gently squeeze out the water. Combine the cream cheese with the spinach in a bowl. Season with black pepper.
- Remove the mushrooms from the oven and tip out any liquid. Put a spoonful of the cream cheese mixture into each mushroom, spreading firmly across the base of the mushrooms. Sprinkle with the goat's cheese. Season again with black pepper. If you are preparing these in advance, you can pop these into the fridge until needed, otherwise return them to the oven for a further 5–8 minutes until golden.
- Make the dressing by putting all the ingredients in a jar, seal and shake to combine.
- Place the salad leaves on each plate. Sprinkle over the bacon, red onion and avocado.
- When the mushrooms are cooked, place them on top of the salad. Finish with a drizzle of salad dressing before serving.

Mushroom 'risotto'

This is a rice-free risotto, made instead with cauliflower rice. You will be surprised how great this tastes. It is very easy to prepare and is delicious topped with a sprinkling of grated Parmesan.

SERVES 4

NUTRITIONAL INFORMATION PER SERVING
253 KCALS
13.4G FAT
10.1 NET CARBOHYDRATES
6.5G PROTEIN

10g dried porcini mushrooms
Knob of butter or ghee
1 onion, finely chopped
400g mixed mushrooms (shiitake, oyster, chestnut, wild, etc.), diced or quartered
300g uncooked cauliflower rice (p146)
200ml white wine or vegetable stock
Handful of fresh tarragon, chopped
Zest of 1 lemon
2 spoonfuls of full-fat crème fraîche
Salt and freshly ground black pepper
Handful of tarragon or parsley, chopped (to garnish)
Parmesan, to serve

- Soak the porcini mushrooms as directed on the pack. This usually takes 20 minutes. Retain the fluid to add it to the stock.
- Heat the butter in a saucepan. Add the onion and fry until translucent. Stir in the fresh and soaked mushrooms.
- Add the cauliflower rice and stir in, ensuring that the rice is completely covered in the butter mixture.
- Add the wine and stir thoroughly. The wine will evaporate and will flavour the rice.
- After 10 minutes, the cauliflower rice should be tender (but not too soft as it should still have a little bite to it). Season with salt and pepper. Add the tarragon and lemon zest. Stir in the crème fraîche.
- Serve immediately, garnished with the chopped herbs and a grating of Parmesan.

Low-carb chilli

This chilli can be made in advance and frozen. It does not use kidney beans as these are not permitted on the LCHF way of eating.

SERVES 6

NUTRITIONAL INFORMATION PER SERVING
373 KCALS
23.7G FAT
10.7G NET CARBOHYDRATES
25.9G PROTEIN

Olive oil, for frying
1 red onion, finely chopped
1 star anise
2 cloves of garlic, crushed
1 red pepper, deseeded and diced
2 sticks of celery, chopped
1–2 chillies, to taste, chopped
150g chorizo, chopped (optional)
500g beef mince
400g tin chopped tomatoes
80g chestnut mushrooms, chopped
1–2 tsp chilli powder, to taste
2 tsp paprika
1 tsp ground cumin
2 tsp dried marjoram
2 tsp dried oregano
2 tbsp tomato purée
2 squares of dark chocolate (at least 85% cacao content)
Salt and freshly ground black pepper

- Heat the oil in a saucepan and fry the onion and star anise until the onion starts to soften.
- Remove the star anise and add the garlic, red pepper and celery, and cook for 5 minutes stirring, regularly.
- Add the chillies and chorizo, and cook for a further 2 minutes.
- Add the beef mince and cook until browned.
- Tip in the tomatoes. Half-fill the tin with cold water and swirl around, then pour this into the pan.
- Add the mushrooms, spices, herbs, tomato purée and chocolate. Season to taste.
- Allow to simmer gently for 20 minutes. The longer the cooking time, the thicker the chilli. If it is too thick, you can add more water.
- Serve with cauliflower rice (page 146) or Parmesan tacos (page 224).

Haddock, egg and Gruyère bake

This is such a quick and easy dish, and perfect for a comforting supper.

SERVES 6

NUTRITIONAL INFORMATION PER SERVING
421 KCALS
30.5G FAT
2.1G NET CARBOHYDRATES
29.7G PROTEIN

400g haddock fillets, skinned and roughly chopped
2 hard-boiled eggs, halved or quartered
200ml full-fat crème fraîche
150ml full-fat milk
125g Gruyère cheese, grated
2 tsp English mustard (optional)
50g pork scratchings, finely ground
50g Parmesan cheese, grated
Salt and freshly ground black pepper

- Preheat the oven to 180°C/gas mark 4.
- Put the haddock and hard-boiled eggs in a 20cm square ovenproof dish.
- In a bowl, mix the crème fraîche, milk, Gruyère and mustard. Season to taste. Spoon this over the egg and haddock mixture.
- Mix the pork scratchings and Parmesan together, season well and sprinkle over the crème fraîche mixture.
- Bake for 20 minutes until the haddock is cooked through.

Chicken schnitzel

If you are feeling a bit stressed, grab your rolling pin or tenderising hammer and bash your chicken breasts to make these tasty chicken schnitzels. Kids love them.

SERVES 4

NUTRITIONAL INFORMATION PER SERVING
250 KCALS
10.5G FAT
0.43G NET CARBOHYDRATES
34.7G PROTEIN

400g chicken breasts
50g pork scratchings, crushed
50g Parmesan cheese, grated
2 tsp paprika
1 tsp dried parsley
½ tsp dried oregano
1 egg, beaten
Coconut oil or butter, for frying
Salt and freshly ground black pepper

- Now here is the fun bit! Place the chicken breasts on a chopping board. You can butterfly them if you wish by cutting them in half through the breast. Using a tenderising hammer, bash the chicken until flattened. You may want to cut the resulting pieces into smaller pieces, especially if you are serving to children.
- In a bowl, mix the pork scratchings, Parmesan, paprika, parsley and oregano together. Season to taste.
- In a separate bowl, add the beaten egg.
- Dip the chicken into the egg before coating in the pork scratching mixture.
- I prefer to fry the escalopes in a frying pan, but you can cook them in the oven (180°C/gas mark 4 for 20 minutes).

Chorizo chicken pot

I love the flavour of chorizo, and combined with chicken and sun-dried tomatoes it is heaven. I eat this with steamed vegetables (cavolo nero is my absolute favourite). This recipe also works really well in the slow cooker – cook on low for 6–7 hours.

SERVES 6

NUTRITIONAL INFORMATION PER SERVING
286 KCALS
12.2G FAT
11.5G NET CARBOHYDRATES
30G PROTEIN

1 tsp coconut oil
2 red onions, chopped
2–3 cloves of garlic, to taste, roughly chopped
2 red peppers, deseeded and sliced
3 chorizo sausages, sliced
500g chicken pieces (breast, leg or thigh)
2 tbsp paprika
400ml chicken stock
400g tin chopped tomatoes
3 tsp homemade sun-dried tomato paste (see p250) or tomato purée
1 tsp dried oregano
½ tsp dried marjoram
Small handful of parsley, chopped
30g black olives (optional)
Salt and freshly ground black pepper

- Preheat the oven to 180°C/gas mark 4.
- Heat the oil in a frying pan or chef's stock pan over a medium heat (I use a stock pot that can be transferred to the oven).
- Add the onions, garlic, red peppers and chorizo, and cook for 5 minutes.
- Add the chicken and cook until browned.
- Add all the remaining ingredients, season to taste and simmer gently for 5 minutes.
- Remove from heat and transfer to an ovenproof dish. Cover with a lid or foil and cook in the oven for 25 minutes. Serve with steamed green vegetables.

Shepherd's pie

Kids love this and you can add lots of veggies in the beef mixture or even as your topping. Unlike the traditional potato-topped pie, this is topped with cauliflower mash, which dramatically cuts the carb count. This recipe can be frozen before baking in the oven.

SERVES 6

NUTRITIONAL INFORMATION PER SERVING
333 KCALS
22.5G FAT
6.7G NET CARBOHYDRATES
24.4G PROTEIN

1 tsp coconut oil
1 red onion, chopped
2 cloves of garlic, finely chopped
500g lamb mince (use beef if you prefer)
75g chestnut mushrooms, diced
1 stick of celery, diced
2 tsp yeast extract (make sure it is sugar-free)
1 tbsp tomato purée
200ml beef bone broth or stock
1 bay leaf
2 thyme sprigs
1 tsp paprika, plus extra for sprinkling
Salt and freshly ground black pepper

For the mash
1 large head of cauliflower (about 300g) cut in florets
25g butter
100g mature Cheddar cheese, grated

- Preheat the oven to 180°C/gas mark 4.
- To make the cauliflower mash, put the cauliflower in a steamer and cook until soft.
- Meanwhile, heat the oil in a large frying pan and fry the onion for 1–2 minutes, then add the garlic and mince. Cook until browned, then add the mushrooms and celery.
- Dissolve the yeast extract and tomato purée in the stock, then add it to the mince. Add the bay leaves, thyme and paprika, and season to taste.
- Cook for 20 minutes until tender and reduced to the desired consistency.
- Mash the steamed cauliflower. Add the butter and two-thirds of the cheese. Mix thoroughly.
- Put the mince in a deep 20cm square ovenproof dish and spoon the mash over the top. Be careful not to overfill the dish. Press the mash down gently using a fork. Top with the remaining cheese and a sprinkling of paprika. Bake for 15–20 minutes until golden.

Stuffed rata peppers

These can be made in advance. If you want to get ahead of the game, why not double up the ratatouille and keep some in the freezer for a quick and easy meal? If you want to do this, follow the recipe below, but only cook for a few minutes so that the vegetables remain firm – that way you won't end up with a soggy mess when you reheat.

SERVES 4
VEGETARIAN

NUTRITIONAL INFORMATION PER SERVING
380 KCALS
26.7G FAT
12.8G NET CARBOHYDRATES
17.8G PROTEIN

2 red peppers
250g halloumi cheese, sliced
Olive oil or coconut oil, to drizzle

For the ratatouille
1 tsp coconut oil or butter
1 red onion, sliced
2–3 cloves of garlic, to taste, roughly chopped
1 red pepper, deseeded and diced
1 courgette, diced
1 aubergine, diced
3 tomatoes, diced
2 tbsp sun-dried tomato paste (p250) or tomato purée
1 tsp dried oregano (or small handful of fresh, finely chopped)
1 tsp dried parsley (or small handful of fresh, finely chopped)
½ tsp paprika
Salt and freshly ground black pepper

- Preheat the oven to 180°C/gas mark 4.
- Cut the red peppers in half from top to bottom and scoop out the centre. Place on a baking tray, cut-sides up.
- To make the ratatouille, melt the oil in a deep saucepan over a medium heat. Add the onion, garlic and diced red pepper. Cook for 2 minutes.
- Add the courgette and aubergine, and cook until softened. Add the tomatoes, tomato paste, herbs and paprika. Season to taste.
- Cook gently on the hob for 5 minutes until the vegetables soften – don't overcook, as there is nothing worse than a slimy ratatouille.
- Remove the ratatouille from the heat, spoon into the halved peppers and top with the halloumi. Drizzle with a little oil.
- Bake for 15–20 minutes until golden. Serve with a green salad.

Italian stuffed chicken

This is my son's favourite; if your children like pizza, they will love this.

SERVES 4

NUTRITIONAL INFORMATION PER SERVING
286 KCALS
13.4 FAT
6.1 NET CARBOHYDRATES
34G PROTEIN

4 chicken breasts
4 tbsp tomato purée or homemade sun-dried tomato paste (see p250)
1 red onion, finely sliced
4 slices of ham or pepperoni
Handful of baby leaf spinach
100g mature Cheddar or mozzarella, grated
2 tsp dried oregano
Salt and freshly ground black pepper

- Preheat the oven to 180°C/gas mark 4.
- Cut the chicken breasts almost in half, creating a pocket so that you can stuff the chicken.
- Spread the inside of the chicken with a little tomato purée, then add the onion, ham, spinach and cheese. Secure the pockets with cocktail sticks.
- Place the breasts on a baking dish, ideally so that they are touching.
- Spread the tops of the chicken breasts with the remaining tomato purée and finish with a sprinkling of cheese. Add the oregano and season to taste.
- Bake for 25–30 minutes until the chicken is cooked. Serve with a green salad.

Moussaka

Traditionally, this is made with lamb mince, but I don't think anyone is going to worry if you prefer to use beef.

SERVES 4

NUTRITIONAL INFORMATION PER SERVING
402 KCALS
32G FAT
8G NET CARBOHYDRATES
18.9G PROTEIN

2 aubergines, cut lengthways into 1cm thick slices
Olive oil, for frying
1 red onion
2 cloves of garlic, crushed
400g lamb mince
400g tin chopped tomatoes
3 tsp tomato purée
2 tsp dried mint
2 tsp ground cinnamon
Butter, for frying
300ml full-fat crème fraîche
50g Parmesan cheese, grated, plus extra for sprinkling
Salt and freshly ground black pepper

- Preheat the oven to 180°C/gas mark 4.
- Put the aubergines on kitchen paper and sprinkle with a little salt. Set aside.
- Meanwhile, heat a little oil in a frying pan and cook the onion and garlic. Add the lamb mince and cook until browned.
- Add the tomatoes, tomato purée, mint and cinnamon, and cook for a further 2–3 minutes.
- Shake off the salt and fry the aubergine slices in a frying pan with a little butter. Fry for 2 minutes, drain on kitchen paper and set aside.
- Place a layer of mince in a 20cm square ovenproof dish, followed by a layer of aubergines. Finish with a layer of mince.
- Finally, mix the crème fraîche with the cheese and pour over the mince. Finish with a sprinkling of Parmesan and bake for 30–40 minutes until golden and bubbling.

Creamy fish pie

A very simple, comforting dish, and a family favourite. You can prepare this in advance, ready to pop in the oven when you get home from work.

SERVES 6

NUTRITIONAL INFORMATION PER SERVING
598 KCALS
50G FAT
3.8G NET CARBOHYDRATES
26.9G PROTEIN

200g cauliflower
200g broccoli
450g selection of fish pieces (you can buy fish pie mix)
200g prawns
400ml double cream
100g Cheddar cheese, grated
Small handful of chopped parsley
50g butter
½ tsp mustard powder
Salt and freshly ground black pepper

- Preheat the oven to 180°C/gas mark 4.
- Cut the cauliflower and broccoli into florets and steam until soft.
- Meanwhile, put the fish and prawns in a casserole dish. Season to taste.
- Combine the cream, cheese and parsley, and pour over the fish.
- When the cauliflower and broccoli are cooked, mash them with the butter and mustard. Season to taste.
- Spread the mash on top of the fish and smooth over. Bake for 30 minutes until golden on top. Serve with steamed green vegetables.

Healthier Fast Food

This chapter is full of your favourites, all given a healthy low-carb makeover. Fill your freezer with these recipes so that you are creating your own frozen ready meals. These will be much healthier and, in the long-run, will save you money and time.

Southern fried chicken

If you love Southern fried chicken, try this recipe. Much healthier than any shop or fast-food concoction! It is also really nice cold and makes a great option for packed lunches.

SERVES 6

NUTRITIONAL INFORMATION PER SERVING
273 KCALS
16G FAT
2.3G NET CARBOHYDRATES
27.9G PROTEIN

For the spice mix
150g ground almonds or coconut flour
4 tsp paprika
1 tsp dried parsley
3 tsp chicken seasoning (ensure sugar free)
1 tsp oregano
½ tsp tarragon
1 tsp thyme
1 tsp garlic powder
½ tsp onion powder
½ tsp celery salt
Generous seasoning of black pepper

1 egg, beaten
500g chicken pieces (can be drumsticks, thighs or breasts)

- Preheat the oven to 190°C/gas mark 5.
- To make the spice mix, mix all the ingredients together and put them in a large dish.
- Put the beaten egg in a dish.
- Now for the messy bit: dip the chicken pieces into the egg, then coat in the spice mix, ensuring they are evenly covered.
- These are oven cooked, so you want them to crisp up evenly. To do this, lay the chicken on a wire rack before placing this onto a baking sheet. If your oven allows, you can use your grill pan and place it straight into the oven. The idea is to allow the heat and air to circulate all around the chicken, ensuring an even and crisp cook.
- Cook for 20–30 minutes, depending on the size of the chicken pieces until golden and cooked through.

Tandoori chicken

There is something deeply satisfying about flinging around herbs and spices when cooking, and it is a great way to get the family's attention as the flavours start to waft around the house.

SERVES 6

NUTRITIONAL INFORMATION PER SERVING
365 KCALS
22.3G FAT
7.2G NET CARBOHYDRATES
31.6G PROTEIN

1 tsp ground coriander
1 tsp ground cumin
3–4 tsp curry powder or garam masala, to taste
2 tsp ground turmeric
1 tsp ground cinnamon
2–3 tsp paprika, to taste
2.5cm piece of ginger, peeled and grated
1–2 chillies, to taste, finely chopped
2–3 cloves of garlic, crushed
Zest and juice of 1 lemon
Dash of olive oil
300ml coconut cream
1 red onion, finely chopped
700g chicken pieces (drumsticks, thighs or breasts)

- In a food processor, whizz the spices with the garlic, zest and lemon juice, a dash of olive oil and the coconut cream.
- Place the onion and chicken pieces in a freezer bag and pour over the spice mixture. Tie the top of the bag and combine thoroughly. For the best flavour, leave to marinate for a few hours in the fridge.
- When ready to cook, preheat the oven to 200°C/gas mark 6. Place the chicken in a baking dish and cook for 40 minutes.

Slow-cooked lamb curry

Lamb can be quite tough, and to counteract this, this recipe is designed to be slow cooked, either in a low-temperature oven or, if you have one, a slow cooker.

SERVES 6

NUTRITIONAL INFORMATION PER SERVING
338 KCALS
20.6G FAT
10.5G NET CARBOHYDRATES
25.8G PROTEIN

For the curry paste
3cm piece of ginger, peeled
3–4 cloves of garlic
1–3 chillies, to taste
1–2 tbsp olive oil
Small handful of coriander leaves
1 tbsp garam masala (or use my sugar-free curry mix on p252)
½ tsp ground cumin
2 tsp ground turmeric

1 tsp coconut oil or olive oil
1 large red (or 2 medium) onions, chopped
1 red or yellow pepper, deseeded and sliced
500g lamb, diced
400g tin chopped tomatoes
200ml beef or bone stock
100g coconut cream
Juice of 1 lime

- Start by making the curry paste. In a food processor, add the ginger, garlic, chillies, oil, half the coriander leaves, the garam masala, cumin and turmeric. Whizz to form a paste. Set aside (store in the fridge or freeze until needed).
- If you are using an oven rather than a slow cooker, preheat it to 140°C/gas mark 1.
- Heat the oil in a large frying pan. Add the onion and red or yellow pepper and cook for 2 minutes until softened.
- Add the lamb and brown it, then add the curry paste, tomatoes and beef stock. Simmer for 10 minutes, then transfer to a slow cooker and cook on low for 6 hours, or place in a casserole dish with lid, or a roasting tray covered in foil, and cook for 3 hours in the oven.
- Just before serving, stir in the coconut cream, the remaining coriander leaves and give it a squeeze of lime. Serve on a bed of cauliflower rice (see p146).

Chicken fajita salad

Forget the wraps, this is far nicer and low carb! If you like things spicy you could add some chopped fresh chilli to the seasoning.

SERVES 4

NUTRITIONAL INFORMATION PER SERVING
226 KCALS
17.5G FAT
8.6G NET CARBOHYDRATES
4.5G PROTEIN

500g chicken breasts, cut into strips
Drizzle of coconut oil or olive oil
1 large red or yellow pepper, deseeded and sliced

For the fajita seasoning
2 tsp chilli powder
2 tsp garlic powder
3 tsp paprika
2 tsp dried oregano
1 tsp ground cumin
2 tsp onion powder
1 tsp dried parsley
Salt and freshly ground black pepper

For the salad
150g mixed leaf salad
16 cherry tomatoes, halved
½ cucumber, diced
2 avocados, diced
Extra-virgin olive oil

- To make the fajita seasoning, mix all the ingredients together.
- Place the chicken strips in a bowl and add some of the fajita seasoning – use half the mix if you want it mild, more if you want a bit more kick. Stir well until coated.
- Gently heat the oil in a frying pan. Add the chicken and keep it moving until it cooks evenly and starts to turn white.
- Add the red or yellow pepper and continue to cook until the chicken is cooked through – the timing will depend on the thickness of the chicken, but it should not take more than 10 minutes.
- While the chicken is cooking, prepare the salad by mixing all the vegetables together in a serving bowl, then drizzle with a little oil.
- When the chicken is cooked, transfer it to a serving dish and serve with the salad.

Salmon fingers

Kids love fish fingers, but don't buy the processed supermarket variety. These homemade ones are far tastier and healthier. Get the kids to help you make them! These can be prepared in advance and frozen.

SERVES 6

NUTRITIONAL INFORMATION PER SERVING
331 KCALS
23.5G FAT
0.12G NET CARBOHYDRATES
29.1G PROTEIN

75g pork scratchings, crushed
50g Parmesan cheese, grated
1 tsp dried parsley
1 tsp dried oregano
½ tsp onion salt
Zest of 1 lemon
Salt and freshly ground black pepper
1 egg, beaten
500g skinless salmon fillets

- Preheat the oven to 180°C/gas mark 4. Line a baking tray with baking parchment.
- Put the pork scratchings in a bowl and add the Parmesan, parsley, oregano, onion salt and lemon zest. Season with salt and pepper to taste and combine well.
- In a separate bowl, add the beaten egg.
- Place the salmon fillets on a chopping board and use a sharp knife to cut each fillet in half lengthways into thick fingers.
- Dip the fish fingers into the beaten egg, then into the dry mixture. Place onto the prepared baking tray.
- Bake for 15–20 minutes until golden. Serve with homemade ketchup (see p246).

Lamb koftas

These spicy meatballs are great served with a variety of Indian dishes, or taste great for a packed lunch with a salad, or even cooked on skewers on a barbecue.

SERVES 4 (MAKES 12 BALLS)

NUTRITIONAL INFORMATION PER SERVING
330 KCALS
23.3G FAT
4.2G NET CARBOHYDRATES
25G PROTEIN

500g lamb mince
1 tsp ground cumin
2 tsp paprika
1 tsp ground turmeric
2 tsp ground coriander
1 tsp ground cinnamon
1 tsp chilli powder
1 chilli, finely chopped
1 red onion, very finely chopped
Small handful of coriander leaves, finely chopped
Salt and freshly ground black pepper
2 tbsp coconut oil, melted, or olive oil

- Place the mince in a large bowl and break it up.
- Add all the remaining ingredients and mix thoroughly until evenly combined.
- Form into 12 balls and place on a tray lined with baking parchment. Refrigerate for 30 minutes.
- When ready to cook, you can either fry, oven cook (180°C/gas mark 4 for 15–20 minutes) or barbecue on skewers.

Low-carb chicken curry

I am a bit of a curry addict. I do like them to pack a bit of a punch, so adjust the seasoning to suit your own palate. This recipe uses curry powder or blends, but check your preferred spice blends as some may have added sugar!

SERVES 4

NUTRITIONAL INFORMATION PER SERVING
366 KCALS
21.1G FAT
11G NET CARBOHYDRATES
29.4G PROTEIN

3cm piece of ginger, peeled
3–4 cloves of garlic
1–2 chillies, depending on taste and strength
2 tbsp melted coconut oil or olive oil, plus extra for frying
Small handful of coriander leaves
1 heaped tbsp sugar-free medium curry powder (see p252)
3 tomatoes
1 red onion, chopped
1 red or yellow pepper, deseeded and sliced
400g chicken breasts, diced
200ml hot water or chicken stock
80g baby leaf spinach
1 heaped tbsp almond butter
100g coconut cream
Small handful of coriander, chopped
Zest of 1 lime

- In a food processor, add the ginger, garlic, chillies, oil, coriander, curry powder and tomatoes. Whizz to form a paste. Set aside (store in the fridge or freeze until needed).
- Heat a little oil in a frying pan over a medium heat and cook the onion and red or yellow pepper for 2–3 minutes to soften, then add the chicken and cook until it has turned white (but still pink in the middle). Stir in the paste, then add the hot water or chicken stock.
- Simmer over a low heat for 20 minutes. Ten minutes before serving, add the spinach, almond butter, coconut cream, coriander and lime zest. The spinach leaves will need to be stirred into the curry carefully; once warm they will soften completely. Serve either on its own or with cauliflower rice (see p146).

Grain-free chicken Kiev

A pet hate of mine is savoury foods containing unnecessary sugar. Kievs are no exception. Most shop-bought Kievs contain added sugar. I like to use my own frozen garlic butter, which I store in the freezer in thick slices. Don't worry if you don't have any frozen garlic butter; you can make it with chilled butter instead.

SERVES 4

NUTRITIONAL INFORMATION PER SERVING
620 KCALS
49G FAT
1.3G NET CARBOHYDRATES
43G PROTEIN

4 skinless chicken breasts (about 400g)

For the garlic butter
3–4 cloves of garlic, to taste, crushed and chopped
150g butter, softened
Small handful of finely chopped parsley
Zest of ½ lemon
Salt and freshly ground black pepper

For the crumb mixture
100g pork scratchings, finely ground
50g Parmesan, grated
1 tsp paprika
2 tsp dried parsley
2 tsp dried oregano
1 tsp onion granules
1 egg, beaten

- Start by making the garlic butter. Mix the garlic, butter, parsley and lemon zest together and season to taste. Place a sheet of clingfilm on your worktop and plop the butter mixture in the centre. Wrap to form into a sausage shape and either freeze if making beforehand, or chill in the fridge while you prepare the chicken crust.
- To make the crumb mixture, put the pork scratchings in a bowl with the Parmesan, paprika, parsley, oregano and onion granules and season to taste. Combine well.
- In a separate bowl, add the beaten egg.
- Place the chicken on a chopping board. Use a sharp knife to make a deep pocket in the breasts, making sure you don't cut right the way through the chicken!
- Remove the garlic butter from the fridge or freezer. Cut it into thick chunks and place 1 or 2 chunks into each of the chicken pockets. You need to ensure the chicken is sealed – you can use wooden cocktail sticks for this, although dipping it into the egg and crumb mixture will provide a protective coating to prevent the butter leaking out.
- Dip the chicken into the beaten egg, then the crumb mixture. Place onto a baking tray lined with baking parchment. You can pop these in the fridge to chill until you are ready to cook.
- Bake at 180°C/gas mark 4 for 20–25 minutes until golden.

Flower's 'fat head' pizza

I love this pizza. It is my adaptation of the brilliant 'Fat Head Pizza', which is admired in the world of low carb. You start off making a large pizza, salivating, thinking of consuming the whole lot in one go, but despite the thin crust and innocent looks, this pizza is not for the faint-hearted. It seriously fills you up. I can manage two slices and then I am full. It can also be eaten cold – perfect for packed lunches and snacks. You can also freeze the bases.

MAKES 2 BASES (8 SLICES PER BASE)

NUTRITIONAL INFORMATION PER SLICE (WITHOUT TOPPING)
155 KCALS
12.3G FAT
1.6G NET CARBOHYDRATES
8.5G PROTEIN

250g mozzarella or Cheddar cheese, grated
100g full-fat cream cheese
2 eggs, beaten
200g almond flour or ground almonds
½ tsp chilli powder
½ tsp garlic powder
1 tsp dried oregano
Salt and freshly ground black pepper

- Place the cheese and cream cheese in a bowl and pop it in the microwave for 1 minute to soften, as this makes it easier to form into a dough.
- Remove the bowl from the microwave and stir in all the remaining ingredients. This will form a wet dough – similar to a wet scone mix. Form into a ball and cut into two equal pieces.
- Preheat the oven to 180°C/gas mark 4.
- Place a large sheet of baking parchment on your worktop. Place the dough in the centre of the sheet. Place another sheet of parchment on top of the dough and press down with your hands and knuckles until the dough is about 1cm thick. This is the easiest way to form the base without getting sticky hands and worktop!
- Place the whole lot, including the parchment, onto a baking sheet. Remove the top sheet of parchment. Repeat with the second base.
- Bake for 15 minutes until the bases start to go golden on top. Top with your chosen toppings, then return to the oven for a further 8–10 minutes until bubbling and golden.

Cauliflower pizza base

This is very popular with low-carb, sugar-free and low-calorie dieters. You can use broccoli or finely grated courgette in place of the cauliflower – both work well.

MAKES 2 PIZZA BASES

NUTRITIONAL INFORMATION PER BASE (WITHOUT TOPPING)
302 KCALS
25G FAT
7G NET CARBOHYDRATES
10.8G PROTEIN

1 cauliflower head (about 200g), cut into florets
180g full-fat cream cheese
1 egg
Salt and freshly ground black pepper

- Place the cauliflower in a food processor and whizz until it resembles couscous. If you don't have a food processor, you can grate the cauliflower instead.
- Place the cauliflower in a bowl and pop it in the microwave for 4 minutes on full power. If you prefer not to use a microwave, you can fry the cauliflower in coconut oil for 5–10 minutes. Allow to cool before adding the cream cheese and egg. Season to taste. Cut the 'dough' into two equal pieces.
- Preheat the oven to 180°C/gas mark 4.
- Place a large sheet of baking parchment on your worktop. Place the dough in the centre of the sheet. Place another sheet of parchment on top of the dough and press down with your hands and knuckles until the dough is about 1cm thick. This is the easiest way to form the base without getting sticky hands and worktop!
- Place the whole lot, including the parchment, onto a baking sheet. Remove the top sheet of parchment. Repeat with the second base.
- Bake for 15 minutes until the bases start to go golden on top. Top with your chosen toppings, then return to the oven for a further 8–10 minutes until bubbling and golden.

Healthy Barbecues

When it is barbecue season, we can all be tempted to eat more processed foods, but you don't have to. You can create your own fantastic, healthy recipes, giving family favourites a healthy twist. If you fancy savoury nibbles, you can make your own flavoured nuts, kale or Parmesan crisps (see the Savoury Snacks section). It doesn't only have to be barbecue season to enjoy these recipes! All of them can be cooked on the hob or in the oven.

Simple baked trout

This is a very easy way to cook fresh fish and is really delicious. You can use this recipe with any whole fish.

SERVES 2

NUTRITIONAL INFORMATION PER SERVING
228 KCALS
7.1G FAT
2.1G NET CARBOHYDRATES
36.3G PROTEIN

1 tablespoon butter
Small handful of fresh herbs (a mix of parsley, thyme and dill),
   finely chopped
2 whole trout (about 250g each), cleaned and bones removed
1 lemon, sliced, plus extra lemon juice, for drizzling
Olive oil, for drizzling
Freshly ground black pepper

- Mix the butter and herbs together in a bowl to form a herby butter.
- Put each trout on a piece of buttered foil almost double the size of the trout. Drizzle a little lemon juice over the fish.
- Stuff the cavity of the trout with herby butter and a slice or two of lemon. Add 1–2 dessertspoons of cold water around the fish. Drizzle with a dash of oil and season with black pepper.
- Wrap the foil tightly and securely around each trout. When ready to cook, pop on a medium heat rack on the barbecue. Cook for 20–25 minutes until the fish is tender and flaking.

Beef burgers

These are traditional beefburgers – so easy to make and far tastier than shop-bought varieties. You can serve these with a LCHF/keto bun or, as I prefer, with just a salad and homemade dressing. Delicious!

SERVES 6

NUTRITIONAL INFORMATION PER SERVING
112 KCALS
3.7G FAT
3.1G NET CARBOHYDRATES
16.3G PROTEIN

1 onion, finely chopped
1 clove of garlic, crushed
400g beef mince
1 egg, beaten (optional)
Salt and freshly ground black pepper

- Put the onion, garlic and beef mince in a large bowl and mix thoroughly.
- Add a little beaten egg (if using) if the mixture looks a little dry, and season to taste.
- Mix thoroughly and form into six balls – these should be firm but moist. Use the palm of your hand to flatten the balls into burger patties.
- You can place them in the fridge until you are ready to cook, or freeze them in layers (separate the burgers with layers of parchment to prevent the burgers sticking together).
- Barbecue, grill, oven cook or fry until cooked through. Serve on a bed of salad with a dollop of homemade mayonnaise (see p248).

Variation: If you like your burgers slightly spicy, why not add some chopped chillies, coriander, cumin and paprika to the burger ingredients before mixing. For an added indulgence, add some chopped smoky bacon.

Slow-cooked spiced chicken

I have found that the best (and safest) way of cooking large pieces of chicken on the barbecue is to slow cook them in a low oven first. You simply finish off for 5 minutes on the barbecue to get that special flavour without destroying the chicken! This recipe requires at least 3 hours of marinating time. It uses chicken breasts, but you can use legs or thighs if you prefer.

SERVES 4

NUTRITIONAL INFORMATION PER SERVING
190 KCALS
4.8G FAT
0.93G NET CARBOHYDRATES
30.6G PROTEIN

3 tsp paprika
2 tsp chilli powder
1 tsp garlic powder
1 tsp onion powder
1 tsp dried thyme
500g skinless chicken breasts/pieces
1 tbsp chilli oil, plus extra for drizzling
Salt and freshly ground black pepper

- Mix the spices, flavourings and thyme together in a bowl.
- Place the chicken breasts/pieces on a chopping board and rub with the oil, then the spices, ensuring they are evenly coated. Season.
- Put the chicken in a freezer bag or lidded container. Seal and refrigerate for at least 3 hours or overnight.
- Preheat the oven to 150°C/gas mark 2.
- Place the chicken breasts in a baking dish, drizzle with a little more oil and cover with foil. Cook for 30–40 minutes until cooked through.
- Remove from the oven and place immediately on the barbecue for 5 minutes. Serve on a bed of salad.

Moroccan-style kebabs

Kebabs can be made in advance – these certainly benefit from marinating for a number of hours before cooking.

MAKES 8 KEBABS

NUTRITIONAL INFORMATION PER KEBAB
211 KCALS
16.7G FAT
5.1G NET CARBOHYDRATES
9.4G PROTEIN

2 tsp paprika
1 tsp ground cumin
1 tsp ground turmeric
2 tsp ground cinnamon
1 tsp allspice
1 tsp ground cardamom
1 tsp ground ginger
Small handful of coriander
2 chillies (remove seeds if you don't want it too hot)
2 cloves of garlic
2 tbsp olive oil
400g lamb loin, diced
3 red onions, cut into wedges
Freshly ground black pepper

- Put all the spices and coriander in a food processor with the chillies, garlic and oil, and whizz to form a paste.
- Put the lamb in a freezer bag with the spice paste, making sure the lamb is evenly coated. Secure the bag and refrigerate overnight. If you are using wooden skewers, leave these to soak in water.
- When you are ready to cook, bring the lamb to room temperature.
- Thread the lamb cubes and onion wedges onto eight skewers. Do not discard the remaining paste as you can brush this over the lamb as it is cooking.
- Place on the barbecue and turn regularly until evenly cooked, brushing with paste as they cook.

Baked herby salmon

Some people don't like strong flavours with salmon as they can overpower the delicate flavour of the fish, but I adore this herby salmon, which is ideal for preparing in advance.

SERVES 2

NUTRITIONAL INFORMATION PER SERVING
361 KCALS
25.2G FAT
6G NET CARBOHYDRATES
26.4G PROTEIN

Small handful of basil leaves
Small handful of dill
Juice of 1 lemon
1 tbsp olive oil
Butter, for greasing
1 red onion, sliced
2 salmon fillets (about 125g each)

- Put the herbs, lemon juice and oil in a processor and whizz until combined.
- Grease a piece of foil with butter and add the onion. Place the salmon fillets on top of the onion and spread the herby marinade over the salmon.
- Wrap the salmon tightly and securely in the foil, making sure the edges are sealed.
- Place the parcel over a medium heat on the barbecue and cook for 10–20 minutes, depending on the size of the fillets, until the fish flakes easily.

Barbecued tandoori chicken

You will need to plan in advance as the chicken needs to marinate for a few hours or overnight to make the most of the favours.

SERVES 4

NUTRITIONAL INFORMATION PER SERVING
233 KCALS
7.9G FAT
6.6G NET CARBOHYDRATES
32.7G PROTEIN

For the marinade
1 tsp ground coriander
1 tsp cayenne pepper
1 tbsp garam masala
2 tsp curry powder
2 tsp turmeric
2–3 tsp paprika
1 onion, finely chopped
2–3 cloves of garlic, crushed
2.5cm piece of ginger, peeled and grated
Zest and juice of 1 lemon
Dash of olive oil
100g full-fat natural Greek yoghurt

500g pieces of chicken (use breasts, thighs or legs)

- To make the marinade, mix all the ingredients together in a bowl.
- Put the chicken pieces in a large freezer bag. Pour in the marinade and combine thoroughly, then seal the bag. Leave to marinate in the fridge for a few hours.
- When ready to cook, place on the barbecue and turn regularly to ensure an even cook. Serve on a bed of cauliflower rice (page 146) or with a salad.

Chilli and lemongrass chicken kebabs

This is a great simple supper if you want to plan ahead and enjoy some free time away from the kitchen. Marinate the chicken while soaking the skewers in water overnight or for a few hours before needed. It is easy to prepare – just serve with various salads.

MAKES 8 KEBABS

NUTRITIONAL INFORMATION PER KEBAB
101 KCALS
3.9G FAT
0.6G NET CARBOHYDRATES
15.9G PROTEIN

2 tbsp olive oil
1 lemongrass stalk
1–2 chillies, to taste (remove the seeds if you don't want it too hot)
2–3 cloves of garlic
2cm piece of ginger, peeled
Small handful of coriander leaves
Juice and zest of 1 lime
500g chicken breasts, diced

- A food processor will make your life so much easier with this recipe. Simply add all the ingredients, apart from the chicken, and whizz to form a paste. If you don't have a food processor, finely chop the ingredients and combine well (or use a pestle and mortar).
- Place the mixture in a bowl or freezer bag. Add the chicken and marinate overnight or for 3–4 hours before preparing. At the same time, soak eight skewers (if you are using wooden ones) as this prevents them from burning.
- When ready to cook, thread the chicken pieces onto the skewers – you could alternate each chicken chunk with a cherry tomato, courgette slice or wedge of red pepper.
- Place the kebabs on the barbecue and turn regularly until evenly cooked through. Serve with a lovely salad – perfect, yet so simple!

Marinated king prawn skewers

If you are using wooden skewers, remember to soak them for several hours before you use them to prevent them from burning.

MAKES 6 SKEWERS

NUTRITIONAL INFORMATION PER SKEWER
97 KCALS
8.6G FAT
0.4G NET CARBOHYDRATES
4.5G PROTEIN

18 king prawns, deveined and peeled
1–2 chillies, finely chopped
3–4 cloves of garlic, to taste, finely chopped
1 tbsp rice malt syrup or honey (optional)
Zest and juice of 1 lime
4 tbsp extra-virgin olive oil
Small handful of parsley, chopped
Freshly ground black pepper

- Place the prawns in a freezer bag.
- In a jug, combine all the remaining ingredients and pour into the freezer bag. Seal, making sure all the prawns are coated in the marinade. Leave to rest for at least 1 hour.
- When ready to barbecue, thread three prawns onto each skewer. Brush with any remaining marinade and cook on the barbecue for 3–4 minutes on each side until done.

Sides and Sauces

You will find a range of side dishes and sauces here that can help enhance your main meals.

Cauliflower rice

Cauliflower rice is really popular for those following low-carb diets. Surprisingly, it does not taste overpoweringly like cauliflower, but instead has a light flavour. The consistency is similar to couscous. There are two ways I cook this – one is in the microwave and the other is to sauté. Alternatively, you can steam or place whole florets on a baking tray and roast them before zapping them in a food processor – however, I have never opted for these as I find the sauté and microwave options really easy.

SERVES 4

NUTRITIONAL INFORMATION PER SERVING
39 KCALS
0.4G FAT
4.8G NET CARBOHYDRATES
2.8G PROTEIN

1 whole cauliflower

- Cut the leaves and stalks off the cauliflower, then cut into florets.
- Place the florets in a food processor and pulse for a few minutes until the cauliflower resembles rice. If you don't have a food processor you can grate the cauliflower, but it is messy and time-consuming.

Microwave cooking
- When ready to cook, put the cauliflower in a lidded container, without any water, and pop into the microwave. Cook on full power for 5–8 minutes, depending on your microwave, stirring halfway through to ensure an even cook.
- Fluff up with a fork and serve immediately.

Sauté cooking
- Heat a little butter or coconut oil in frying pan. Add the cauliflower and toss gently over a medium heat for 5–8 minutes until heated through and softened. Serve immediately.

Top tip! Whizz up a few cauliflowers at a time and place the uncooked processed cauliflower rice into freezer bags. You can use this from frozen – just add to a frying pan and cook through.

Curried cauliflower rice

Add a little kick to your cauliflower rice with some Indian spices. If you are using your favourite curry powder, check the ingredients to make sure there is no added sugar.

SERVES 4

NUTRITIONAL INFORMATION PER SERVING
82 KCALS
3.8G FAT
6.7G NET CARBOHYDRATES
3.4G PROTEIN

1 whole cauliflower
1 tbsp butter or coconut oil
1 small red onion, finely chopped
2 cloves of garlic, crushed
1 chilli, finely chopped
1 tsp ground turmeric
1 tbsp sugar-free curry powder (see p252)

- Cut the leaves and stalks off the cauliflower, then cut into florets.
- Place the florets in a food processor and pulse for a few minutes until the cauliflower resembles rice. If you don't have a food processor you can grate the cauliflower, but it is messy and time-consuming.
- Heat the butter in a frying pan. Stir in the onion, garlic, chilli and spices, then add the cauliflower. Stir gently over a medium heat for 5–8 minutes until heated through and softened. Serve immediately.

Cauliflower mash

This is a good staple to add to your LCHF menus. This mash is very easy to make, but I think it really benefits from butter and grated cheese, but the choice is yours! You can also add various herbs, garlic, cream cheese, or even cream, to make your own flavour combinations. If you like, you can swap the cauliflower for broccoli for a more nutritious and probably less smelly option, as long as you don't mind green mash!

SERVES 4

NUTRITIONAL INFORMATION PER SERVING
114 KCALS
7.7G FAT
3.3G NET CARBOHYDRATES
5G PROTEIN

300g head of cauliflower
1 tbsp butter
50g mature Cheddar cheese, grated (optional)
Salt and freshly ground black pepper

- Cut the leaves and stalks off the cauliflower, then cut into florets.
- Steam the cauliflower until soft, then put it in a bowl and mash until soft.
- Stir in the butter and cheese, and mash until creamy. Season to taste.

Variation ideas: This recipe uses a head of cauliflower, but if you are in a hurry you can use pre-packed cauliflower rice, available from supermarkets, and microwave until cooked. Other mash alternatives include sweet potato mash, roasted pumpkin mash or butternut mash. These are all much higher in carbs than cauliflower mash, so use sparingly.

Cauliflower and broccoli cheese

You can use this basic cheese sauce recipe and create your own recipes – I love leeks in cheese sauce, especially when served with roasted gammon. This is also nice with bacon, fish and beef mince to make your own lasagne (I use aubergine slices instead of pasta sheets – see p88) or a moussaka (see p115).

SERVES 4

NUTRITIONAL INFORMATION PER SERVING
612 KCALS
58G FAT
4.2G NET CARBOHYDRATES
11.7G PROTEIN

150g cauliflower
150g broccoli
350ml double cream
75g mature Cheddar cheese, grated
Freshly ground black pepper

- Cut the cauliflower and broccoli into florets and steam until just soft.
- Put the cream in a saucepan and heat gently. When warm, add the cheese and season to taste. Stir over a low-medium heat until the cheese has melted, making sure the heat is not too high or the sauce will stick to the bottom of the pan and burn. Taste and adjust by adding more cheese or seasoning to suit.
- Put the cauliflower and broccoli in an ovenproof dish and pour over the sauce. You can eat this as it is, or if you prefer, you can add more grated cheese and place it under the grill until golden and bubbling.

Wilted kale with garlic and lemon

This is a lovely side dish, with a great flavour. I have made a meal out of this by adding some grated Parmesan and serving with sliced cooked chicken and lardons. Delicious.

SERVES 4

NUTRITIONAL INFORMATION PER SERVING
83 KCALS
6.6G FAT
1.8G NET CARBOHYDRATES
3.3G PROTEIN

25g butter
2–3 cloves of garlic
Zest and juice of 1 lemon
100ml stock or water
350g kale, shredded
Salt and freshly ground black pepper

- Melt the butter in a frying pan and add the garlic and lemon zest.
- Add the stock, then the kale. Cover with a lid and cook for 5–8 minutes.
- Remove the lid and season to taste. Finish with the lemon juice. Stir well until combined. Serve immediately.

Cauliflower bites

These are really tasty and make a lovely side dish with a salad, steamed vegetables or even a variety of curries, or they can be served as a starter – lovely with some crumbled blue cheese over the top.

SERVES 4

NUTRITIONAL INFORMATION PER SERVING
316 KCALS
24.8G FAT
3.3G NET CARBOHYDRATES
17.2G PROTEIN

200g cauliflower, cut into small florets
75g pork scratchings, finely ground
2 tsp paprika
1 tsp dried oregano
50g Parmesan cheese, finely grated
3 tbsp crème fraîche
1 large egg
Salt and freshly ground black pepper

- Preheat the oven to 180°C/gas mark 4.
- Blanch the cauliflower in a pan of boiling water for 2 minutes. Drain well.
- Meanwhile, put all the dry ingredients in a bowl and season with salt and pepper. Combine well.
- Put the crème fraîche in a separate bowl and mix in the egg.
- Dip the cauliflower florets in the crème fraîche mixture, then roll them in the dry mixture.
- Place on a lined baking tray. Bake for 10–15 minutes until golden.

Creamy sauces

Creamy sauces are really easy with this way of eating. You can make a simple sauce by adding pesto, mustard or peppercorns to cream.

Peppercorn sauce

This is lovely with steak, but it can also be used with other meats or as a base for a pork or chicken dish.

SERVES 6

NUTRITIONAL INFORMATION PER SERVING
262 KCALS
26.8G FAT
1.2G NET CARBOHYDRATES
0.83G PROTEIN

1 tsp butter
½ small onion, very finely diced
1 tbsp brandy
300ml double cream
2 tbsp peppercorns, crushed
Salt

- Melt the butter in a frying pan and cook the onion until soft. Pour in the brandy and reduce slightly for 5 minutes.
- Add the cream and peppercorns. Cook to your desired thickness. Season with salt to taste. Serve immediately.

Creamy mushroom sauce

This sauce goes with anything. It is also nice as a vegetarian dish or starter: use large chestnut mushrooms and add a handful or two of spinach and a small handful of chopped thyme.

SERVES 6

NUTRITIONAL INFORMATION PER SERVING
257 KCALS
26.9G FAT
1.3G NET CARBOHYDRATES
1.2G PROTEIN

1 tsp butter
½ small onion, very finely chopped
1 clove of garlic, crushed
75g mushrooms (sliced, halved or quartered)
300ml double cream
Salt and freshly ground black pepper

- Melt the butter in a frying pan and cook the onion and garlic for 5 minutes.
- Add the mushrooms and cook until slightly soft.
- Add the cream and season to taste. Cook to your desired thickness. Serve immediately.

Hollandaise sauce

A lovely buttery sauce, perfect on poached eggs over thick slices of bacon (my low-carb version of eggs Benedict!).

SERVES 4

NUTRITIONAL INFORMATION PER SERVING
362 KCALS
39G FAT
0.26G NET CARBOHYDRATES
1.8G PROTEIN

175g butter, melted
2 egg yolks
1 tbsp white wine vinegar
Salt and freshly ground black pepper

- Melt the butter, but do not let it burn or brown. You can do this in a microwave or saucepan.
- Half fill a saucepan with water and place a bowl on top, making sure the base doesn't touch the water. Bring to a medium heat.
- Place the egg yolks in the bowl along with the vinegar, and whisk in the butter over the heat (it must not be too hot) for a few minutes until you get a thick sauce. Season to taste.

The Savoury Baker

One of the most common questions I get when clients go on to this way of eating, is how to make bread. It is quite funny as we all start out missing bread, but within a few months, that craving disappears. Low-carb bread must be made grain free and yeast free (as yeast feeds off sugar, starch and grain), so it's quite a challenge. If you are after the same taste, texture and smell of a fresh loaf, then you may be disappointed.

I make bread occasionally, but to be honest I find it too filling, so one slice is often enough. The internet is full of keto/low-carb bread recipes. Some are better than others, but one thing they all have in common is expensive ingredients! Purple bread can happen with some brands of psyllium husk powder; green bread can happen when the baking powder reacts to the sunflower seeds. It is very much trial and error. Cloud bread is very popular. For me, one of the best recipes is keto bread from www.dietdoctor.com.

White low-carb bread

Nothing is going to recreate the fresh white loaf or the flavour exactly, as we are not using wheat or yeast. This is more like a savoury cake in texture, but it is very good toasted and topped with sugar-free jam (page 244) or chocolate spread (page 241). My seeded bread (page 157) is more savoury.

CUTS INTO 14 SLICES

NUTRITIONAL INFORMATION PER SLICE
228 KCALS
19.4G FAT
2.1G NET CARBOHYDRATES
8.6G PROTEIN

110g butter
6 large eggs, beaten
250g ground almonds
40g coconut flour
1 tsp baking powder
½ tsp xanthan gum
½ tsp salt
½ tsp onion granules (optional)
½ tsp garlic granules (optional)
20g mixed seeds

- Preheat the oven to 160°C/gas mark 2. Line a 900g loaf tin with baking parchment.
- Melt the butter in a saucepan, then add the eggs. Beat well before adding all the remaining ingredients, but not the mixed seeds.
- Combine well, then pour into the prepared loaf tin and top with the mixed seeds.
- Bake for 45 minutes until golden and crusty on the outside.
- Leave to cool on a wire rack. Store in an airtight container for up to 5 days. (This loaf can also be frozen.)

Chestnut and flax seed bread (sugar/grain/yeast free)

I have experimented with lots of LCHF bread recipes (including many that have come out purple thanks to psyllium husk). I like the dense nutty flavour, like a dark rye bread, but if you are looking for a light, white loaf, this isn't for you!

MAKES 1LB LOAF (ABOUT 8 THICK SLICES)

NUTRITIONAL INFORMATION PER SLICE
243 KCALS
21G FAT
1.5G NET CARBOHYDRATES
9.4G PROTEIN

50g butter or 1 tbsp coconut oil
4 eggs
120g ground flax seeds
60g chestnut flour, ground almonds or almond flour (or coconut flour)
1 tsp baking powder
1 tsp cream of tartar
30g mixed seeds

- Preheat the oven to 180°C/gas mark 4. Line a 400g loaf tin with baking parchment.
- Beat the butter until soft; if using coconut oil, melt and place in a bowl.
- Add the eggs and 3 tablespoons of cold water and beat well.
- Mix in all the remaining ingredients, combining well.
- Transfer to the prepared loaf tin and bake for 30–40 minutes until golden and firm.
- Leave to cool on a wire rack before slicing.

Top tip! I don't eat much bread, so once cold, I slice this and freeze it. When I want a slice of bread, I take one out, toast it or leave it to defrost if I prefer a sandwich.

Low-carb savoury bagels

These are as near as you are going to get when it comes to bagels. They are best cut in half and lightly toasted.

MAKES 8 BAGELS

NUTRITIONAL INFORMATION PER BAGEL
158 KCALS
11.6G FAT
2G NET CARBOHYDRATES
8.8G PROTEIN

6 large eggs
80g soured cream
½ tsp baking powder
½ tsp paprika
½ tsp onion granules
¼ tsp garlic powder
60g ground almonds
½ tsp dried oregano
40g coconut flour
2 tsp butter or coconut oil, for greasing
Salt and freshly ground black pepper

- Preheat the oven to 180°C/gas mark 4.
- Beat the eggs with the soured cream, then add all the remaining ingredients, except the butter, stirring well.
- Grease a doughnut pan (I use a silicon doughnut tray) before pouring the mixture into each ring.
- Bake for 25–30 minutes until the bagels are golden on top. Leave to cool on a wire rack and store in an airtight container for up to 5 days.

Quick-and-easy toasted English muffin

This is a recipe I discovered on Facebook. I have tried to find who originally wrote the recipe, but no luck. It is a 2-minute muffin made in the microwave, so it is perfect if you are in a hurry and want comfort food. It does need to be toasted and is really good with butter and some sugar-free jam (page 242).

MAKES 1 MUFFIN

NUTRITIONAL INFORMATION PER SERVING
527 KCALS
44G FAT
5.6G NET CARBOHYDRATES
20.2G PROTEIN

15g butter
45g ground almonds
10g coconut flour
½ tsp baking powder
1 egg

- Put the butter in a mug or ramekin and melt in the microwave for 20 seconds.
- Remove and stir in all the remaining ingredients.
- Leave to rest for 5 minutes to thicken, then cook in the microwave for 1½ minutes.
- Remove the muffin from the mug or ramekin – the easiest way to do this is to run a knife around the edge and then flip it onto a plate.
- Slice the muffin in half. Toast and serve with butter and sugar-free jam.

Cheese, bacon and onion pinwheels

I used to make these when I was a child. Sunday was a day of baking and our roast dinner. The oven always had to be full, so it was packed with cakes and savouries for the week ahead. These pinwheels were a firm favourite – it's so lovely to be able to recreate a low-carb version.

MAKES 8 PINWHEELS

NUTRITIONAL INFORMATION PER PINWHEEL
328 KCALS
24.2G FAT
4.8G NET CARBOHYDRATES
18.7G PROTEIN

For the dough
180g grated mozzarella cheese
30g full-fat cream cheese
150g ground almonds
40g coconut flour
1 large egg, beaten

6 rashers of bacon, diced
1 onion, diced
75g mature Cheddar cheese, grated
5g Parmesan cheese, grated
2 tsp dried oregano

- Preheat the oven to 180°C/gas mark 4.
- Start by making the dough. Melt the cheese and cream cheese in the microwave for 1 minute.
- Stir in all the remaining dough ingredients and combine well. Allow to stand for 5 minutes.
- Place a large sheet of baking parchment on your worktop. Have another sheet of the same size to hand.
- Place the dough in the centre of the baking parchment and top with the other sheet of parchment, so that the dough is sandwiched between the two.
- Use your hand or a rolling pin and smooth the dough into a rectangle about 1cm thick. Set aside to rest.
- Cook the bacon and onion in a sauté pan.
- Sprinkle the dough with the Cheddar and Parmesan, then the onion and bacon pieces. Finish with the oregano.
- Hold the edges of the baking parchment and use to help roll the dough on the longest edge, into a large sausage.
- Cut into 8 slices, 2–3cm thick. Place on a lined baking tray. Bake for 20–30 minutes until golden. Remove from the oven and leave to cool on a wire rack.

Grain-free low-carb crackers

The secret is to make these crackers quite thin and get them as crispy as possible without burning them! Times are approximate, as much depends on the efficiency of your oven and the thickness of your dough!

MAKES 12 CRACKERS

NUTRITIONAL INFORMATION PER CRACKER
119 KCALS
10.2G FAT
0.8G NET CARBOHYDRATES
5.4G PROTEIN

125g mature Cheddar or mozzarella cheese, grated
75g cream cheese
1 egg
100g ground almonds
½ tsp chilli powder
1 tsp dried oregano
1 egg, beaten, for eggwash (optional)
Sprinkling of Parmesan cheese (optional)
Salt and freshly ground black pepper

- Preheat the oven to 190°C/gas mark 5.
- Place the cheese and cream cheese in a bowl and pop in the microwave for 1 minute to soften, as this makes it easier to form into a dough.
- Remove from the microwave and add the remaining ingredients except the egg for eggwash and Parmesan. Season with salt and pepper and combine well. This will form a wet dough, similar to a wet scone mix.
- Form the dough into a ball. Place a large sheet of baking parchment on your worktop, add the ball of dough in the centre of the parchment. Place another sheet of parchment on top of the dough and press down with your hands.
- This is the easiest way to form the base without getting sticky hands and worktop!
- Press into a rectangle or square shape using your hands and knuckles. The dough should be about 0.5–1cm thick.
- Place the whole thing, including the parchment paper, on a baking sheet, then peel off the top sheet of parchment.
- Using a knife, gently score out the crackers. This makes it easier to break them into perfect squares or rectangles once baked. Brush with eggwash and sprinkle with Parmesan, if liked.
- Bake for about 10 minutes, until golden on top.
- Remove from the oven, flip over and peel away the baking parchment. This helps to get the base of the crackers as crispy as the top.
- Pop back into the oven for a further 8–10 minutes until golden.
- Leave to cool on a wire rack before breaking/cutting into crackers.

Low-carb sausage rolls

This basic and versatile recipe uses a grain-free pastry. I use a similar recipe as a base for pizza and also for grain-free crackers. It is a bit sticky to handle, so arm yourself with some good-quality baking parchment. Be careful when buying sausage meat, as most contain sugar and grains. Check the ingredients or speak to your butcher. You can also buy sausages and use these instead of sausage meat if you prefer, but remember to remove the skin or you will end up with a very tough skin to bite into!

MAKES 8 SAUSAGE ROLLS

NUTRITIONAL INFORMATION PER SAUSAGE ROLL
392 KCALS
33G FAT
2.5G NET CARBOHYDRATES
20G PROTEIN

250g Cheddar or mozzarella cheese, grated
120g ground almonds
1 tsp paprika
½ tsp chilli powder
1 egg, beaten
400g good-quality sausage meat
1 tsp dried thyme
1 tsp dried sage
1 tsp dried parsley
1 egg, beaten, or full-fat milk, for brushing
2 tbsp sesame seeds
Salt and freshly ground black pepper

- Place the cheese in a bowl and pop into the microwave to melt slightly for 30–45 seconds.
- Stir in the ground almonds, paprika and chilli powder. Add the egg and season to taste. Combine to form a dough. Leave to rest in the fridge for 10 minutes, as this helps to firm it up.
- Preheat the oven to 180°C/gas mark 4.
- You may find the dough difficult to roll, so what I do is place it on a large sheet of baking parchment, top this with another large sheet of baking parchment, then use a rolling pin or my hands to flatten the dough into a rectangle roughly 1cm thick.
- In a bowl, mix the sausage meat with the thyme, sage and parsley. Season well.
- Shape the sausage meat into one or several sausages (whatever is easier to handle) and pop them onto the dough, leaving enough dough to comfortably roll over the top of the sausage(s).
- Brush the pastry with a little beaten egg or milk, then wrap the pastry over the top of the sausage(s), pressing down firmly. Cut into sausage rolls.
- Brush with the remaining egg and sprinkle with the sesame seeds.
- Bake for 20 minutes until golden.

Cheese straws

A low-carb variation of cheese straws. They are great for packed lunches. They are also nice spread with yeast extract and grated cheese before they are folded.

MAKES 15 STRAWS

NUTRITIONAL INFORMATION PER STRAW
151 KCALS
11.6G FAT
1.7G NET CARBOHYDRATES
8.7G PROTEIN

For the dough
180g grated mozzarella cheese
30g full-fat cream cheese
150g ground almonds
40g coconut flour
20g Parmesan cheese, grated
1 tsp chilli powder
½ tsp mustard powder
1 large egg

50g mature Cheddar cheese, grated
1 tsp chilli flakes (optional)
2 tsp dried oregano
1 egg, beaten, or full-fat milk, for brushing
1–2 tsp sesame seeds (optional)

- Preheat the oven to 180°C/gas mark 4.
- Melt the mozzarella and cream cheese in the microwave for 1 minute.
- Stir in all the remaining dough ingredients and combine well. Allow to stand for 5 minutes.
- Place a large sheet of baking parchment on your worktop. Have another sheet of the same size to hand. Place the dough in the centre of the baking parchment and top with the other sheet of parchment, so the dough is sandwiched between the two.
- Use your hand or a rolling pin and smooth the dough into a 1cm thick rectangle.
- Cover the dough with the Cheddar and sprinkle with the chilli flakes, if using, and the oregano.
- Fold in half and roll again into a rectangle.
- Cut into 15 ribbons about 1–1.5cm wide. Place on a baking tray lined with baking parchment.
- Brush with beaten egg or milk. Sprinkle with the sesame seeds, if you like.
- Bake for 20–25 minutes until golden. Leave to cool on a wire rack.

The Sugar-free Baker

I love baking. There is something wonderfully homely and comforting about smelling cakes baking in the oven, and for me, the whole process of baking is a massive stress-buster. Whatever life throws at me, baking a cake, while listing to good music, never fails to make me smile.

Even though we are following a sugar-free, low-carb lifestyle, there is no reason why we can't still indulge in a delicious cake, biscuit or treat. The key is to choose the right ingredients, and, that horrible word – MODERATION!

SWEETENERS

Please read the information on sweeteners in the Sugar chapter (page 18). It is for this reason you will find all the recipes state the quantities for xylitol and erythritol, but not for stevia, as it is very much down to personal taste and the brand of stevia you use.

FLOURS

Remember that flours are carbohydrates and the aim is to keep the carbs as low as possible. Low-carb alternatives are nut flours, and these work very well. You can swap most flours for ground almonds, almond flour or a nut flour – a combination of hazelnut flour and ground almonds works really well in cakes. I like to use either all ground almonds/almond flour or a 60/40 combination of almond and hazelnut. Some people find a combination of coconut flour and almond flour to be the best combination with a ratio of three parts almond flour to one part coconut flour, which also works well.

You can also grind your own nuts to make your own nut flours, which is by far the healthiest option. I use my NutriBullet to do this, but you can also use a food processor. Don't over-process or you will end up with a nut butter instead of a flour! Store in the freezer to prevent them going rancid.

Coconut flour

If swapping to coconut flour, remember to adjust the liquid, as coconut flour absorbs almost 10 times its volume, so if you are not careful you could end up with a very dry cake! I have found I get the best results when baking with coconut flour if I use one egg and two tablespoons of liquid (milk, water, buttermilk or Greek yoghurt) per 30g of coconut flour. As coconut flour is very absorbent, you will need to use less coconut flour in recipes, roughly half. It does take some getting used to. The texture of cakes is always different with coconut flour (grainier and dry), but you can make quite good cakes – it just takes a little practice.

ALWAYS sieve coconut flour before using it, as it can clump up in the packaging.

Almond flour and ground almonds

Almond flour is much finer and does give superior results in cakes, but to be honest, I use ground almonds all the time as they are far cheaper and the results are almost as good. Sukrin is the best brand of almond flour I have found in the UK.

Cooking times with nut flours

Cooking times may vary when using nut flours, as the mixture is a different consistency. Use my timings as a guide and check every 5 minutes after this time if your cakes are not yet cooked. I prefer to bake cakes on a low temperature for longer, so most of my recipes reflect this.

Please note when using nut flours that they may still be very crumbly until they are completely cold. This is particularly the case when baking cookies, which harden as they cool, so try not to move them too much until they are completely cold.

Chocolate torte

This is seriously good and would pass muster at a dinner party. It is lush with a dollop of cream and some raspberries – mind you, for me, everything is lovely with cream and raspberries!

SERVES 8

NUTRITIONAL INFORMATION PER SERVING
378 KCALS
31G FAT
9.3G NET CARBOHYDRATES
11.3G PROTEIN

1 tsp butter, for greasing
275g dark chocolate (at least 85% cacao content)
5 eggs, separated
150g erythritol or xylitol (or stevia, to taste)
140g almond flour or ground almonds
Cocoa, for sprinkling (optional)

- Preheat the oven to 180°C/gas mark 4. Grease and line a 20cm round cake tin.
- Melt the chocolate in a heatproof bowl over a pan of gently simmering water, making sure the base of the bowl doesn't touch the water, or use a microwave (this takes seconds).
- In a clean bowl, whisk the egg whites until they form soft peaks.
- In a separate bowl, whisk the egg yolks with the erythritol until light and fluffy.
- Carefully fold half the egg whites into the egg yolks, then the chocolate, then the rest of the egg whites – carefully so as not to knock out any air. Finally, fold in the almond flour.
- Pour the mixture into the prepared tin. Bake for 30 minutes. Turn off the oven and keep the cake in there for a further 10 minutes. The torte will be cracked on top, but this is as it should be. Sprinkle with cocoa, if liked.

Lemon shortbread biscuits

This is a lovely almond shortbread recipe, suitable for those on a low-carb diet. It's a really easy recipe, which gives you something to nibble on with your cuppa when you are feeling the need!

MAKES 8 BISCUITS

NUTRITIONAL INFORMATION PER BISCUIT
303 KCALS
28.7G FAT
1.9G NET CARBOHYDRATES
7.2G PROTEIN

125g butter, melted
225g almond flour or ground almonds
55g erythritol or xylitol (or stevia, to taste)
1 tsp gelatine powder
Zest of 2 lemons

- Preheat the oven to 190°C/gas mark 5. Line a baking tray with baking parchment.
- Melt the butter in a saucepan and pour onto the almond flour.
- Combine with the remaining ingredients and allow to rest for 10 minutes to stiffen up a little.
- Form into eight balls and press down onto the prepared tray.
- Bake for 10–15 minutes until golden. The biscuits will be slightly moist when they come out of the oven. They harden up as they cool, but they are quite crumbly, so avoid the temptation to move them around too much until they are cold. If they are too moist, turn the temperature down and pop them back into the oven for a further 5 minutes.
- Store in an airtight container for up to 5 days.

Chocolate muffins

I have been experimenting a lot with chocolate muffin recipe combinations. I wanted the muffins to have a very light, fluffy sponge, as often LCHF and sugar-free muffins can be a bit dense and dry if overcooked. These were perfect, and the general opinion is that people would be hard pushed to know that they were made without grains or sugar. Try them for yourself!

MAKES 12 LARGE MUFFINS

NUTRITIONAL INFORMATION PER MUFFIN
202 KCALS
17.8G FAT
2.2G NET CARBOHYDRATES
6.5G PROTEIN

100g butter
50g cream cheese
4 large eggs (or weigh eggs to make 250g)
150g ground almonds
60g cocoa or cacao
80g erythritol or xylitol (or stevia, to taste)
1 tsp baking powder

- Preheat the oven to 170°C/gas mark 3. Line two muffin trays with paper cases.
- Put all the ingredients in a mixing bowl and beat until combined, making sure not to overbeat.
- Pour the mixture into the muffin cases and smooth the tops to ensure they rise evenly. Bake for 20 minutes until firm to the touch.
- Turn out on a wire rack to cool before storing in an airtight container for up to 5 days.
- You can decorate the muffins with homemade chocolate ganache (page 189), sugar-free icing (see page 189), melted dark chocolate or thick whipped cream.

Apple and cinnamon Danish rolls

This is a low-carb, grain-free Danish, which tastes the same as a regular Danish and is lovely with a cup of coffee.

MAKES 8 DANISH ROLLS

NUTRITIONAL INFORMATION PER DANISH ROLL
280 KCALS
21.7G FAT
5.4G NET CARBOHYDRATES
12.9G PROTEIN

For the dough
180g grated mozzarella cheese
30g full-fat cream cheese
150g ground almonds
50g coconut flour
30g erythritol or xylitol (or stevia, to taste)
1 tsp sugar-free vanilla extract
1 large egg
2 tsp ground cinnamon

For the filling
40g butter
30g Sukrin Gold (brown erythritol) or you can use erythritol
   or xylitol
2 tsp ground cinnamon (more if you like a rich cinnamon flavour)
1 tsp mixed spice
1 Bramley cooking apple, cored and sliced

- Preheat the oven to 180°C/gas mark 4. Line a baking tray with baking parchment.
- Melt the cheese and cream cheese in the microwave for 1 minute.
- Stir in all the remaining dough ingredients and combine well. Allow to stand for 5 minutes.
- Place a large sheet of baking parchment on your worktop. Have another sheet of the same size to hand. Place the dough in the centre of the baking parchment and top with the other sheet of parchment, so the dough is sandwiched between the two.
- Use your hand or a rolling pin and smooth the dough until it is a rectangle 1cm thick. Allow to rest while you make the filling.
- Melt the butter in a saucepan, then stir in the sweetener, cinnamon and mixed spice. Combine well until the butter and sweetener has melted/dissolved. Add the apple and cook in the butter mixture for a few minutes.
- Peel off the top sheet of baking parchment. Spread the cinnamon and apple slices onto the dough.
- Hold one long edge of the baking parchment and use this to help roll the dough into a large sausage. Cut into 8 slices, 2–3cm thick. Place these onto the prepared baking tray.
- Bake for 30 minutes until golden, then cool on a wire rack. Drizzle with a sugar-free icing if liked (see p189).

Millionaire's shortbread

My mum used to make this for us when we were children: a shortbread base with a thick layer of caramel, topped with chocolate. I wasn't sure how this would turn out, but it is surprisingly good and avoids the cloying sickliness of the original version.

To get a nice golden caramel, opt for Sukrin Gold (a natural brown sugar alternative). White erythritol or xylitol works well and will give a creamy colour caramel. I used 100 per cent dark chocolate, but feel free to use at least 85 per cent to avoid too much sugar.

CUTS INTO 18 SMALL SQUARES

NUTRITIONAL INFORMATION PER SQUARE
416 KCALS
41G FAT
3.6G NET CARBOHYDRATES
5.2G PROTEIN

For the base
200g hazelnuts
100g unsweetened desiccated coconut
100g almond flour or ground almonds
1 tsp baking powder
110g butter
40g erythritol or xylitol (or stevia, to taste)
1 large egg, beaten

For the filling
100g butter
60g erythritol or xylitol (or stevia, to taste)
350g double cream

For the topping
150g very dark chocolate (at least 85% cacao content)
20g coconut oil

- Preheat the oven to 180°C/gas mark 4. Line a 22cm square brownie tin with baking parchment.
- Start by making the base. To make the hazelnut flour, grind the hazelnuts in a NutriBullet or food processor until they resemble flour. Don't over-process or they will turn into nut butter! Do the same with the coconut.
- Mix the flours and baking powder together in a bowl.
- Melt the butter in a saucepan over a low heat. Add the sweetener, combining until dissolved.
- Pour the melted butter onto the dry ingredients, add the beaten egg and combine well to form a wet dough. Transfer the dough to the prepared baking tin and smooth out the top. Bake for 20–25 minutes until golden. Remove from the oven and leave to cool in the tin.
- To make the filling, put the butter and sweetener into a saucepan over a low–medium heat. Melt completely before stirring in the cream. Stir continuously for about 10 minutes until thickened and glossy, making sure the heat isn't too high as it can splutter and bubble and could burn you. Remove from the heat and pour onto the base in the tin. Place in the freezer for about 30 minutes to set.
- Meanwhile, make the topping. Melt the chocolate and coconut oil in a heatproof bowl over a pan of gently simmering water, making sure the base of the bowl doesn't touch the water, or use a microwave (this takes seconds). Pour this over the chilled base. Return to the freezer for a further 30 minutes.
- Remove from the tin and slice into 18 squares. I keep this in the fridge as it benefits from remaining cool.

Nutty bars

These are a cross between a tray bake and cereal bars. They are perfect for packed lunches and lovely to snack on with a cuppa.

MAKES 15 BARS

NUTRITIONAL INFORMATION PER BAR
231 KCALS
20.4G FAT
2.8G NET CARBOHYDRATES
7G PROTEIN

100g mixed nuts, chopped
150g ground almonds
40g flaked almonds
60g very dark chocolate chips (at least 85% cacao content)
70g erythritol or xylitol
60g butter, melted
100g almond butter
2 eggs, beaten

- Preheat the oven to 170°C/gas mark 3. Line a 22cm square tin with baking parchment.
- In a bowl, mix together the nuts, ground almonds, flaked almonds, chocolate chips and sweetener.
- Melt the butter in a saucepan, then stir in the almond butter until it is smooth and lump free. Pour onto the dry mixture. Add the eggs and combine well.
- Pour into the prepared tin, smoothing down the surface. Bake for 20–25 minutes until golden and firm to the touch.
- Remove from the oven and allow to cool completely before cutting into 15 bars. Store in an airtight container for up to 5 days.

Hazelnut and pecan chocolate brownie

A variation of my favourite brownie. This texture is surprisingly light and fluffy. Hazelnut flour is well worth the preparation. I don't buy the hazelnut flour; instead I grind hazelnuts in my NutriBullet or food processor.

CUTS INTO 9 SQUARES

NUTRITIONAL INFORMATION PER SQUARE
347 KCALS
31.1G FAT
3.8G NET CARBOHYDRATES
10.4G PROTEIN

100g butter, softened, plus extra for greasing
60g cream cheese
100g ground hazelnuts
100g ground almonds
70g cocoa or cacao
4 large eggs
100g erythritol or xylitol (or stevia, to taste)
1 tsp baking powder
40g pecan nuts

- Preheat the oven to 160°C/gas mark 2½. Grease and line a 22cm square brownie tin.
- Combine all the ingredients, except the pecans, in a food mixer or mix with a wooden spoon. Pour into the prepared tin.
- Place the pecan nuts randomly into the batter, pressing down so that they are just below the surface.
- Bake for 30–40 minutes until firm in the centre (I prefer to cook over a lower heat for longer as I believe it gives better results).
- Remove from the oven and leave to cool on a wire rack, then cut into 9 squares. Store in an airtight container for up to 5 days.

Chocolate chip bites

My son makes these and often coats them with dark chocolate. They are great as a quick snack or for a child's lunchbox.

MAKES 10 BITES

NUTRITIONAL INFORMATION PER BITE
143 KCALS
11.8G FAT
2.1G NET CARBOHYDRATES
5.6G PROTEIN

2 eggs, beaten
2 tbsp almond butter
60g erythritol or xylitol (or stevia, to taste)
120g ground almonds
1 tsp baking powder
1 tsp sugar-free vanilla extract
40g very dark chocolate chips (at least 85% cacao content)

- Preheat the oven to 180°C/gas mark 4. Line a baking tray with baking parchment.
- Combine the eggs, almond butter and sweetener together, then stir in the ground almonds, baking powder and vanilla. Finally, stir in the chocolate chips.
- Place dollops of the mixture (roughly 1–2 dessertspoons) onto the prepared tray to make 10 bites.
- Bake for 20 minutes until golden, then cool on a wire rack. Store in an airtight container for up to 5 days.

Lemon drizzle cake

Lemon drizzle was one of my dad's favourite cakes. This is a low-carb/grain-free version that is super-moist, even a few days after it has been cooked. This is also lovely with some blueberries mixed into the batter before cooking.

CUTS INTO 10 SLICES

NUTRITIONAL INFORMATION PER SLICE
212 KCALS
18.9G FAT
1.9G NET CARBOHYDRATES
6.8G PROTEIN

100g butter
100g full-fat cream cheese
75g erythritol or xylitol
Zest and juice of 3 lemons
90g ground almonds
40g coconut flour
1 tsp baking power
5 eggs

- Preheat the oven to 160°C/gas mark 2½. Line a 900g loaf tin with baking parchment.
- In a bowl, beat the butter, cream cheese and sweetener together until pale and creamy. Stir in the lemon zest.
- Add the remaining ingredients (except the lemon juice) and combine well. Pour into the prepared tin.
- Bake for 30–40 minutes. After about 20 minutes, when the cake looks slightly golden on top but not quite done, remove it from the oven and pour some lemon juice over it. Pop it straight back into the oven. Do this every 5 minutes until the cake is cooked or you have used up all the lemon juice.
- To check the cake is cooked, insert a knife or skewer into the centre of the cake – it should come out clean.
- Leave to cool completely in the tin (any cake made with almond or coconut flour needs to cool or it can be very crumbly). Store in an airtight container for up to 5 days.

Dark chocolate walnut cake

This is a really rich, dark chocolate cake, peppered with a sprinkle of walnuts to add a little texture. It is really delicious served warm with some extra-thick cream and a handful of berries, or have it cold with a cuppa.

SERVES 10

NUTRITIONAL INFORMATION PER SERVING
332 KCALS
31G FAT
3.2G NET CARBOHYDRATES
7.9G PROTEIN

180g butter
100g erythritol or xylitol
4 eggs
140g ground almonds
1 heaped tsp baking powder
40g sugar-free cocoa or cacao powder
40g walnuts, chopped
40g very dark chocolate chips (95% cacao content)

- Preheat the oven to 160°C/gas mark 2½. Line a 22cm round springform cake tin with baking parchment or use a cake tin liner.
- Put the butter and sweetener in a food mixer and beat until light and fluffy.
- Add all the remaining ingredients and combine well. The resultant batter will be quite thick. Pour into the prepared tin.
- Bake for 30–40 minutes until firm. Remove from the oven and place on a wire rack to cool (or eat while still warm). Store in an airtight container for up to 5 days.

Lemon and blueberry muffins

I was determined to get perfect blueberry muffins with a light, fluffy sponge. They turned out great, and only 2g of carbs per cake!

MAKES 12 MUFFINS

NUTRITIONAL INFORMATION PER MUFFIN
235 KCALS
21.1G FAT
2.4G NET CARBOHYDRATES
7.2G PROTEIN

100g butter
60g cream cheese
80g erythritol or xylitol (or stevia, to taste)
240g almond flour or ground almonds
1 tsp baking powder
4 large eggs (to weigh 240g)
Zest and juice of 2 large lemons
100g blueberries

- Preheat the oven to 180°C/gas mark 4. Line a 12-hole muffin tin with paper cases.
- Put all the ingredients, except for the blueberries and lemon juice, in a food mixer and blend until combined (don't over-blend).
- Fold in the blueberries, then spoon the batter into the muffin cases. Smooth the tops to ensure an even rise.
- Bake for 20 minutes until firm and golden. Remove from the oven and gently pour the lemon juice on top of each cake. Return to the oven for a further 3–5 minutes. Leave to cool in the tin on a wire rack.

Bakewell tart

A family favourite with a sugar-free, low-carb twist! You can top this with flaked almonds as given here, or if you prefer, some sugar-free icing. Use the sugar-free raspberry jam from page 242.

SERVES 10

NUTRITIONAL INFORMATION PER SERVING
494 KCALS
45G FAT
3.7G NET CARBOHYDRATES
14.2G PROTEIN

For the pastry
40g butter, plus extra for greasing
300g ground almonds
75g ground hazelnuts
1 egg, beaten

For the batter
125g butter
100g erythritol or xylitol (or stevia, to taste)
125g almond flour or ground almonds
1 egg, beaten
1 tsp almond essence

2 tbsp sugar-free raspberry jam (page 242)
30g flaked almonds

- Preheat the oven to 180°C/gas mark 4. Grease a 20cm round pie dish.
- Start by making the pastry. Rub the butter into the ground nuts until the mixture resembles breadcrumbs. Add the egg and form into a dough – it will be very crumbly as it has no gluten to hold it together.
- Put the pastry in the pie dish and flatten and spread it using your hands until the base is covered. Try to spread the dough slightly up the side, but if you find this too tricky, don't worry. Bake for 10 minutes.
- Meanwhile, make the batter. Put the butter and sweetener in a bowl and beat until light and fluffy. Add the almond flour, egg and almond essence, and beat well until evenly combined.
- Remove the nut pastry from the oven.
- Spread the jam onto the pastry case (don't be tempted to add more jam as it will bubble up and spill). Pour over the cake batter and smooth the top. Sprinkle with the flaked almonds.
- Bake for 30–40 minutes until golden on top and the sponge springs back when touched. Remove from the oven and leave to cool in the dish. You can coat with sugar-free icing (see p189) if you like. Store in an airtight container for up to 5 days.

Chocolate roulade

This roulade is rich, light and fluffy. If you are not used to dark chocolate, you may find this a little bit bitter as it has a very rich cocoa flavour. This makes a great Christmas log when covered in dark chocolate ganache (see p189).

CUTS INTO 8 SLICES

NUTRITIONAL INFORMATION PER SLICE
239 KCALS
22G FAT
1.7G NET CARBOHYDRATES
6.7G PROTEIN

6 eggs, separated
100g erythritol or xylitol
1 tsp sugar-free vanilla extract
50g cocoa or cacao
250ml double cream
100g fresh raspberries

- Preheat the oven to 180°C/gas mark 4. Line a Swiss roll tin (39x24x2cm) with baking parchment, making sure the paper hangs over the edges a little.
- Put the egg whites in a clean bowl and beat until they form soft peaks.
- In a separate bowl, mix the egg yolks with the sweetener and vanilla until the mixture becomes thick and doubles in size. It is important to spend some time mixing this well. It will have a mousse-like texture. Sift in the cocoa and beat again.
- Stir a spoonful of the egg white into the cocoa mixture to help loosen the mixture. Add the remaining egg whites and very carefully fold in until combined. Don't overmix as you will knock the air out.
- Pour the mixture in the tin and bake for 20 minutes.
- Remove from the oven and lift the cake off the tin, holding onto the baking parchment (do not remove the baking parchment)! Place on the worktop and carefully start rolling from one long end into a roll. Leave to cool.
- While the cake is cooling, whip the double cream, then fold in the raspberries, leaving some raspberries whole and some crushed.
- Carefully unroll the sponge. Don't press down on it or it may split. Carefully spread over the cream filling, then re-roll. Place on a plate ready to serve.
- Because of the filling, this will have to be refrigerated. However, if you opt for a different filling, it should keep well in an airtight container for up to 5 days. You can also freeze the sponge.

Coconut macaroons

These are slightly different from the coconut macarons that are piled high with fluffy coconut. These are more a biscuit and are great on their own or topped with dark chocolate. This recipe is not good with stevia, so use erythritol or xylitol.

MAKES 12 MACAROONS

NUTRITIONAL INFORMATION PER MACAROON
170 KCALS
15.6G FAT
1.6G NET CARBOHYDRATES
2.6G PROTEIN

4 egg whites
300g desiccated coconut
120g erythritol or xylitol

- Preheat the oven to 160°C/gas mark 2½. Line a baking tray with baking parchment.
- In a bowl, whip the egg whites until they are light and fluffy. Gently mix in the desiccated coconut and sweetener.
- Place a spoonful of the mixture onto the tray. Using the back of a dessertspoon, press down on the mixture and spread gently to form a flat circle. Repeat with the remaining mixture to make 12 macaroons.
- Bake for 10 minutes, or until golden. Watch the biscuits carefully as they burn quite quickly!
- Remove from the oven and place on a wire rack to cool. Store in an airtight container for up to 5 days.

Cake frostings and toppings

There are some products on the market to make your own icing, such as Natvia icing, and Sukrin do a nice blend too. Both work well and are great substitutes for icing sugar. I will leave that to you to experiment with. Meanwhile, here are some sugar-free toppings I love, but these may have a more limited shelf life, or have to be kept in the fridge.

You can of course use fresh cream and maybe add a few low-fructose berries to a lovely sponge.

Chocolate ganache

This ganache is really easy to make, but watch the sugar content of the chocolate. Use as high a cocoa content as you can.

250ml cream
200g dark chocolate (at least 85% cacao content), grated

- Put the cream in a saucepan over a medium heat. Heat it gently and don't let it boil. When it is warm, remove it from the heat.
- Stir in the chocolate until it has melted. The mixture will start to thicken and become glossy. Cool before using on a cake or in a dessert.

Lemon cream filling

This is one of my favourite fillings, but it does have to be stored in the fridge. You can also make this in a raspberry flavour by adding 80g fresh or frozen raspberries and omitting the lemon.

120g cream cheese
3 tbsp thick cream or Greek yoghurt
Zest of 1 large lemon
A little milk or lemon juice, if needed

- In a bowl, beat the cream cheese, cream and lemon zest together until well combined. If you prefer a thinner mixture, add a little milk or lemon juice.
- I use this with a little sugar-free lemon curd (p243) to fill a lemon sponge or lemon butterfly cupcakes. It is also lovely with some crushed raspberries.

Easy creamed frosting

A very easy base for any flavoured frosting. Add your flavourings to taste.

200g Greek yoghurt
200g cream cheese
1 tsp sugar-free vanilla extract

- In a bowl, blend all the ingredients together to a smooth, creamy texture.
- Mix in any flavouring you wish. Cocoa, lemon juice, fresh/frozen raspberries or coffee all work well.

Sugar-free Desserts

It is always lovely to have a special dessert after a meal, but they can be packed with unnecessary sugar. No diet is sustainable if we deprive ourselves of certain foods, but the good news for those following an LCHF way of eating is that the desserts are amazing! Just think of all those foods we have been told for years are too full of fat or too rich, which are now free for us to consume, albeit without sugar!

Remember, if you are starting out, you want to limit your berry consumption until your blood sugars have started to stabilise, but there are some great recipes here that will keep you going so you won't miss the berries. I have highlighted the fruit options as higher fructose to remind you all.

Lemon meringue pie

I love this dessert! I use a lot of lemons, because I love the intense citrus flavour and it contrasts so well with the creamy meringue and the crumbly nutty pastry base.

SERVES 8

NUTRITIONAL INFORMATION PER SERVING
523 KCALS
49G FAT
2.8G NET CARBOHYDRATES
15.8G PROTEIN

For the pastry base
150g hazelnuts
150g ground almonds
100g butter
1 egg, beaten

For the lemon filling
100g butter
100g erythritol or xylitol (or stevia, to taste)
Juice and zest of 4 lemons
4 eggs
3 egg yolks

For the meringue topping
3 egg whites
2 tbsp erythritol or xylitol (or stevia, to taste)

- Preheat the oven to 160°C/gas mark 2½.
- Start by making the pastry base. Place the hazelnuts in a NutriBullet or food processor and pulse until fine. Place the ground hazelnuts and ground almonds in a bowl. Rub in the butter using your fingertips. Add the beaten egg and combine until the mixture forms a soft dough. You may need to use your hands for this. Refrigerate for 10 minutes.
- Place the dough between two pieces of parchment paper and spread gently using your hands. Remove the top piece of paper and flip the dough into a flan dish. You will need to gently press the dough into the base and up the side of the dish, spreading it out evenly.
- Bake for 20–30 minutes until the base is golden brown.
- Meanwhile, make the filling. Place a bowl over a pan of simmering water, making sure the base of the bowl doesn't touch the water.
- Put the butter, sweetener, lemon juice and zest in the bowl and heat until the butter has melted.
- Remove from the heat and gradually add the eggs and yolks one at a time, mixing well with a balloon whisk between each addition.
- Return to the heat and continue to whisk until the mixture starts to thicken and become glossy – this can take up to 10 minutes. Pour into the pastry case.
- To make the topping, whisk the egg whites until they are fluffy. Add the sweetener and continue to whisk until firm peaks form. Spread the meringue all over the lemon base.
- Bake for 10–15 minutes at the same oven temperature until the meringue is golden.
- Leave to cool before serving.

Raspberry trifle

This is another family favourite and I make this at least once a month. I put the trifle in individual pots with lids and pop them in the fridge, adding the cream when we are ready to eat them, but you can make this in a large bowl if you prefer.

SERVES 6

NUTRITIONAL INFORMATION PER SERVING
385 KCALS
34.1G FAT
10.9G NET CARBOHYDRATES
7.1G PROTEIN

To make the raspberry jelly

Don't be afraid to make jelly; it is really simple and makes a delicious dessert in its own right. It also has the added benefit of having gelatine, which is great for your bones, nails and hair. I use Great Lakes gelatine powder.

200g frozen raspberries
1 tbsp erythritol or xylitol (or stevia, to taste) (optional)
1 heaped tbsp gelatine powder

- Place the raspberries in a saucepan with 150ml cold water. Heat gently, squashing a few of the raspberries. Add a little sweetener if liked, although personally I don't think it needs anything.
- Stir in the gelatine powder (I don't bother to mix with water first) until it has dissolved into the raspberry liquid, then remove from the heat and pour into a bowl or individual dishes.
- Pop into the fridge to set for 2–3 hours.

To make the custard

Homemade vanilla custard is absolutely heavenly and works brilliantly with this way of eating. Start making the custard when the jelly has set.

4 egg yolks
30g erythritol or xylitol (or stevia, to taste)
30g arrowroot powder
600ml full-fat milk (or use half milk and half double cream)
1 tsp sugar-free vanilla extract
300ml thick or double cream, whipped (for topping)
Raspberries, to garnish

- In a bowl, whisk the egg yolks, sweetener and arrowroot together until the mixture becomes pale and fluffy.
- Meanwhile, heat the milk in a saucepan until it starts to simmer. Remove the milk from the heat and add a little at a time to the egg mixture, whisking continuously.
- When combined, pour back into the saucepan and place over a low heat. Continue to whisk until the custard starts to thicken – it needs to be quite thick, but be careful it does not burn.
- Remove from the heat and allow to cool for 10 minutes, then pour onto the jelly. Refrigerate for 1–2 hours, or until set.
- When ready to serve, top with the cream and garnish with a few raspberries.

No-bake lemon cheesecake

This is one of my family's favourites. We tend to have this as an extra at Christmas as it helps cleanse the palate! I don't use gelatine in this recipe as I find it sets to a nice soft consistency without it.

SERVES 10

NUTRITIONAL INFORMATION PER SERVING
512 KCALS
50G FAT
3.7G NET CARBOHYDRATES
8.6G PROTEIN

300g mixed nuts, (hazelnuts, brazil, almonds, pecan or macadamia)
3 tbsp butter, melted, plus extra for greasing
500g full-fat cream cheese
300g extra thick double cream
Zest and juice of 3 lemons

- Grease a 23cm loose-bottomed round tin.
- Put the nuts in a food processor and blend until they resemble breadcrumbs.
- Put in a bowl and stir in the melted butter.
- Spread the nuts out in the tin, pressing them down to form a solid base. Refrigerate for 30 minutes to set.
- While the base is chilling, mix the remaining ingredients together in a bowl. Pour this onto the chilled base and spread to level. Refrigerate for at least 3 hours to set the filling.
- You can decorate the top of the cheesecake with sugar-free lemon curd (page 243) or some blueberries.

Chocolate custard

This is lovely on its own or to accompany a chocolate pudding such as my Hazelnut and Pecan Chocolate Brownies (page 179).

SERVES 6

NUTRITIONAL INFORMATION PER SERVING
146 KCALS
8.3G FAT
10.1G NET CARBOHYDRATES
6.2G PROTEIN

4 egg yolks
30g erythritol or xylitol (or stevia, to taste)
30g sugar-free cocoa or cacao
30g arrowroot powder
600ml full-fat milk (or use half milk and half double cream)
1 tsp sugar-free vanilla extract

- In a bowl, whisk the egg yolks, sweetener, cocoa and arrowroot together until the mixture turns pale and fluffy.
- Meanwhile, heat up the milk in a saucepan until it starts to simmer.
- Mix the milk into the egg mixture, adding a little at a time and whisking continuously.
- When combined, pour back into the saucepan and place over a low heat.
- Continue to whisk until the mixture starts to thicken. It needs to be quite thick, but be careful it does not burn. Serve hot or cold.

Panna cotta and raspberry jelly layer

These are really easy to make and look quite impressive. They do take a few hours to set, so allow for this.

SERVES 6

NUTRITIONAL INFORMATION PER SERVING
376 KCALS
40G FAT
1.7G NET CARBOHYDRATES
1.2G PROTEIN

For the panna cotta
450ml double cream
2 tbsp erythritol or xylitol (or stevia, to taste)
2 tsp sugar-free vanilla extract (or 2 vanilla pods)
1 heaped tsp gelatine powder (or use 1 sheet, soaked)

- Place the cream in a saucepan and slowly heat. Add the sweetener and vanilla, and combine until the sweetener has dissolved.
- Stir in the gelatine powder (I sprinkle this straight in, but you can mix it with a little water first if you prefer; if you are using sheets, leave them to soak before adding them to the cream). Stir until everything is dissolved.
- Remove from the heat and pour into six glasses. Pop into the fridge to set for 1½–2 hours.
- When the panna cotta is set, prepare the jelly.

For the raspberry jelly
250g frozen raspberries
200ml boiling water
1 tbsp erythritol or xylitol (or stevia), to taste (optional)
1 heaped tsp gelatine powder (or use 1 sheet, soaked)

Mixed berries, to serve

- Place the raspberries in the saucepan and heat over a medium heat.
- Add the boiling water and sweetener, if using. I personally don't think it needs it, but some people prefer a sweeter jelly.
- Add the gelatine powder (I sprinkle this straight in but you can mix it with a little water first if you prefer. If you are using sheets, soak them before adding to the raspberries). Stir until well combined.
- Remove from the heat and leave to cool before pouring onto the panna cotta.
- Refrigerate for 2 hours to set. Top with mixed berries before serving.

Chocolate panna cotta

Wow! I love this and it really is so simple to make. You can claim it is a healthy dessert as it is packed with antioxidants from the rich, dark chocolate as well as gelatine powder to help with your joints, hair and nails. Really, what could be better?

SERVES 6

NUTRITIONAL INFORMATION PER SERVING
398 KCALS
36.7G FAT
9.1G NET CARBOHYDRATES
6.3G PROTEIN

2 tsp gelatine powder
600ml thick double cream
2 tbsp erythritol or xylitol (or stevia, to taste)
150g dark chocolate (at least 85% cacao content)

- Put the gelatine powder in a cup and add about 75ml cold water. Stir well and set aside.
- Meanwhile, heat the cream, sweetener and chocolate in a saucepan over a medium heat. Reduce the heat to low, then stir in the gelatine until combined – I use a balloon whisk to do this.
- Pour into 6 ramekins or glasses. Leave to chill in the fridge for at least 3 hours.
- Serve with thick cream and raspberries.

Strawberry and rhubarb crumble

I love rhubarb – there is nothing nicer than picking fresh rhubarb from the garden and making this delicious dessert. Rhubarb goes well with strawberries, which I add just before popping on the crumble topping.

This recipe is high in fructose and natural sugars, so it should be an occasional treat and only eaten once your blood sugars are stable.

SERVES 8

NUTRITIONAL INFORMATION PER SERVING
369 KCALS
32.6G FAT
4.4G NET CARBOHYDRATES
9.7G PROTEIN

650g rhubarb
75g erythritol or xylitol (or stevia, to taste)
100g strawberries, quartered
75g mixed nuts
200g ground almonds
40g mixed seeds
100g butter

- Preheat the oven to 180°C/gas mark 4.
- Place the rhubarb in a saucepan and add the sweetener and 100ml cold water. Cook gently over a low-medium heat for 5–8 minutes to soften the fruit, then add the strawberries and cook for 10 minutes.
- Pour the fruit into a 20cm square ovenproof dish.
- Place the mixed nuts in a food processor and whizz until they resemble fine breadcrumbs.
- In a bowl, combine the ground almonds, nuts and seeds. Add the butter and rub with your fingertips until the mixture resembles breadcrumbs. Tip this over the fruit base, making sure it is spread evenly.
- Bake for 20 minutes. Serve with a dollop of cream or my homemade custard (page 195).

No-bake chocolate cheesecake

It is really nice to have a sweet, especially when you are starting out on sugar free. I would always opt for erythritol or xylitol – stevia is good, but it can be a bit hit and miss to get the right sweetness for your palate – too much and it can leave a chemical aftertaste.

SERVES 10

NUTRITIONAL INFORMATION PER SERVING
378 KCALS
34.3G FAT
6.8G NET CARBOHYDRATES
8.1G PROTEIN

75g ground almonds
75g hazelnuts, finely chopped
20g sugar-free cocoa powder
20g erythritol or xylitol (or stevia, to taste) (optional)
75g butter, melted, plus extra for greasing
200g cream cheese
200g extra-thick cream
150g full-fat Greek yoghurt, plus extra to serve
150g dark chocolate (at least 85% cacao content), plus extra to decorate

- Mix the ground almonds, hazelnuts, cocoa and sweetener in a bowl. Pour on the melted butter.
- Using the back of a spoon, press down firmly into a 20cm greased spring-form cake tin. Refrigerate while you complete the next phase.
- In a bowl, mix the cream cheese, cream and yoghurt together.
- Melt the chocolate in a heatproof bowl over a pan of gently simmering water, making sure the base of the bowl doesn't touch the water, or use a microwave (this takes seconds). Then stir it into the creamy mixture. Refrigerate until set.
- Grate some dark chocolate on the top and serve with fresh raspberries and a dollop of Greek yoghurt.

Variation: Add a few drops of mint or orange essence to the mixture to create a whole new flavour.

Berry cream meringues

These little meringues can be stored in an airtight container and are great for a quick and easy dessert. Remember, you can adjust the sweetener to your taste, as your palate changes.

SERVES 6

NUTRITIONAL INFORMATION PER SERVING
119 KCALS
9.8G FAT
3.2G NET CARBOHYDRATES
3.2G PROTEIN

3 egg whites
75g erythritol or xylitol (or stevia, to taste)
1 tsp arrowroot
½ tsp white wine vinegar
250ml double cream, whipped
150g mixed berries

- Preheat the oven to 200°C/gas mark 6. Line a baking tray with baking parchment.
- Place the egg whites in a clean bowl and whisk until glossy and soft peaks form.
- Add the sweetener a little at a time and beat to firm peaks. Stir in the arrowroot and vinegar.
- Pipe or spoon the mixture to form 6 rounds.
- Place in the oven and immediately reduce the temperature to 150°C/gas mark 2.
- Cook for 1 hour, then turn the oven off, leaving the meringues inside to cool.
- Remove and place on a wire rack to cool. If the meringues are soft or spongy, leave them in a dry place as they will harden over a period of hours. Store in an airtight container until needed.
- Place the meringues on a serving plate, add a dollop of cream and top with the berries.

Chocolate mousse

This is rich in essential fatty acids, but tastes like a luxury chocolate mousse – perfect! It does not have any sweetener in it – the creaminess of the avocado and cream should be enough – but if you like things sweet, you can use liquid stevia, or new on the block is a fibre syrup by Sukrin, which works out at 5g of carbs per 100g.

SERVES 3

NUTRITIONAL INFORMATION PER SERVING
255 KCALS
23.2G FAT
4.8G NET CARBOHYDRATES
4.4G PROTEIN

1 ripe avocado, mashed
2 tbsp sugar-free cocoa powder (or 60g dark chocolate at least 90% cacao content, melted)
150g double cream
Liquid stevia drops, to taste (optional)

Optional extras (choose one)
A few drops of vanilla, orange or mint extract
1 tsp pure nut butter

- Put all the ingredients, except the sweetener, in a blender and blend until smooth.
- Taste as you go and add sweetener to suit, if using. Mix in your chosen optional extra.
- Pour into individual glasses. Chill, then serve with fresh berries.

Baked egg custard

Egg custard was something my mum would always bake for me when I was feeling poorly. For me, it is the ultimate comfort food.

SERVES 2

NUTRITIONAL INFORMATION PER SERVING
257 KCALS
22.5G FAT
2.1G NET CARBOHYDRATES
11.4G PROTEIN

4 eggs
200ml double cream or full-fat milk
2 tbsp erythritol or xylitol (or a few drops of stevia, to taste)
1 tsp sugar-free vanilla extract (optional)
Finely grated nutmeg or ground cinnamon

- Preheat the oven to 180°C/gas mark 4. Boil the kettle so that you have plenty of hot water.
- In a bowl or jug, beat the eggs with the cream/milk, sweetener and vanilla, if using.
- Pour into ramekins and sprinkle with nutmeg or cinnamon.
- Place in a deep-sided baking tray (I use a brownie tray) and fill the tray with hot water until it comes halfway up the ramekins.
- Bake for 20–25 minutes until firm.

Key lime pie

So lovely, refreshing and tasty. Traditionally, this would have a biscuit base, but I have replaced this with a lovely nutty base and swapped condensed milk for a more natural filling, with added avocado for more essential fatty acids. I don't think this needs any sweetener.

SERVES 10

NUTRITIONAL INFORMATION PER SERVING
427 KCALS
43G FAT
2.8G NET CARBOHYDRATES
6.3G PROTEIN

For the base
200g nuts (I use pecans, walnuts, almonds, Brazils and hazelnuts)
50g butter, melted

For the filling
2 ripe avocados, mashed
Zest and juice of 4 limes
Zest and juice of 1 lemon
180g cream cheese
300g extra-thick double cream
1 tsp gelatine powder (mixed with 75ml water)

- Grease and line a flan dish.
- Start by making the base. Grind the nuts in a food processor.
- Transfer to a bowl and stir in the melted butter. Tip into the prepared flan dish. Use your fingers to press the mixture down evenly. If you can, press around the edge to form a raised side. Refrigerate for 30 minutes.
- To make the filling, whisk all the ingredients together in a bowl using a food mixer until evenly combined. Pour onto the nut base and smooth. Refrigerate for a further 2 hours.
- Decorate with whipped cream and slices of lime, if liked.

Top tip: To get the most juice out of your limes, roll them on a work surface for a few minutes.

Blueberry clafoutis

This takes minutes to prepare and is so lovely when you fancy a dessert. I serve this with a dollop of Greek yoghurt or thick cream while it is still warm. You can replace the blueberries with any other berry or cherries. I use fresh, but you can use frozen as long as the fruits aren't too wet.

SERVES 8

NUTRITIONAL INFORMATION PER SERVING
357 KCALS
33.6G FAT
2.5G NET CARBOHYDRATES
9.4G PROTEIN

Butter, for greasing
100g fresh blueberries
75g erythritol or xylitol (or stevia, to taste)
4 eggs, beaten
Zest of 1 lemon
125ml full-fat milk
300ml cream
1 tsp sugar-free vanilla paste (optional)
150g ground almonds

- Preheat the oven to 180°C/gas mark 4. Grease a flan dish.
- Put the blueberries in the dish.
- Beat the remaining ingredients together and pour over the blueberries.
- Bake for 40 minutes, or until firm and golden.

Chocolate pecan meringue layer cake

Now, when I call this a cake, it really is more of a dessert. It is so decadent, it almost has a pavlova texture, hence why I have popped this into the dessert section. It's one of those cakes you simply have to eat with a cake fork, devouring while enjoying your own private blissed-out moment. This recipe does not work with stevia.

SERVES 10

NUTRITIONAL INFORMATION PER SERVING (WITHOUT FILLING)
447 KCALS
36.5G FAT
7.3G NET CARBOHYDRATES
12G PROTEIN

5 eggs, separated
150g erythritol or xylitol
75ml hot water
350g pecan nuts, plus extra to decorate
1 tbsp sugar-free cocoa
1 tsp sugar-free vanilla extract
4 tbsp Chocolate ganache (page 189) and/or whipped double cream
Chocolate shavings, to decorate

- Preheat the oven to 170°C/gas mark 3. Line three sponge tins with baking parchment.
- In a clean bowl, whisk the egg whites to very stiff peaks.
- In a separate bowl, mix the egg yolks with the sweetener and beat until really light and pale. This can take up to 10 minutes. Add the hot water as you beat.
- Whizz the pecan nuts in a food processor until finely ground. Add to the egg yolk mixture with the cocoa and vanilla.
- Very gently fold the eggy pecan mixture into the egg whites. Spoon the mixture into the tins and spread carefully.
- Bake for 1 hour. Do not open the oven during this time unless you feel the cakes are cooking too quickly. Remove from the oven and place on a wire rack to cool.
- Carefully sandwich the cakes together with chocolate ganache and/or whipped cream. You can also cover the top, but be very careful, as this is a very delicate cake.
- Decorate with chocolate shavings and pecans.

Molten chocolate puddings

My son loves these just out of the oven and served with homemade ice cream or cream. This recipe is for four people, but you can halve the quantities if you want to make less.

SERVES 4

NUTRITIONAL INFORMATION PER SERVING
497 KCALS
42G FAT
6.4G NET CARBOHYDRATES
18.8G PROTEIN

75g butter, plus extra for greasing
75g sugar-free cocoa or cacao powder, plus extra for dusting
120g ground almonds or almond flour
100g erythritol or xylitol
1 tsp sugar-free vanilla extract (optional)
4 eggs
Sugar-free icing (see p189) and berries, to decorate

- Preheat the oven to 180°C/gas mark 4. Grease four 7cm ramekins with butter and dust with cocoa.
- In a mixing bowl, combine all the ingredients together and blend using a food mixer.
- Spoon into the ramekins and smooth the tops. Bake for 12–15 minutes until firm on top.
- Remove from the oven. Run a knife around the sides of the ramekins, then tip the puddings onto plates. Sprinkle with a little sugar-free icing and add a couple of berries for a professional finish!

The Ice-cream Parlour

Ice creams and lollies are seen as a treat, but they can contain anything from 3–6 teaspoons of sugar. It is not just the sugar content that is incredibly worrying, it is the ingredients list. Most read more like a science project than real food. We don't need emulsifiers, caramelised sugar syrups, stabilisers, colourings, locust bean gum, beetroot juice, reconstituted skimmed milk, carrageenan, potato starch, ammonium phosphatides, fructose syrups, palm oils, etc.

At the time of writing, the only ice creams in the UK that are sugar free are WheyHey and Oppo. Both are sweetened with xylitol.

Creamy almond and dark chocolate lollies

My son said that these are very similar to the almond magnums. They are very easy to make, but you have to do these in two stages, so plan in advance. You will need lolly moulds.

MAKES 6 LOLLIES

NUTRITIONAL INFORMATION PER LOLLY
415 KCALS
34.6G FAT
9.8G NET CARBOHYDRATES
12.7G PROTEIN

400g full-fat Greek yoghurt (I use Total)
100g full-fat cream cheese
150g almond butter (or use any nut butter to suit)
2 tbsp erythritol or xylitol (or liquid stevia, to taste)
20g almond flakes, crushed
200g dark chocolate (at least 85% cacao content)
2 heaped tsp coconut oil

- Put the yoghurt, cream cheese, almond butter and sweetener in a blender and whizz until smooth. Fold in the almond flakes and pour into 6 lolly moulds.
- Freeze until solid (this should take 4–5 hours).
- Just before removing from the freezer, melt the chocolate with the coconut oil in a heatproof bowl over a pan of gently simmering water, making sure the base of the bowl doesn't touch the water, or use a microwave for 50 seconds.
- Remove the lollies from the freezer and extract them from their moulds. Cover with the chocolate, then return to the freezer to set (you can place the lollies on a sheet of greaseproof paper or insert the lolly sticks into a piece of polystyrene to hold them upright while they freeze). Once frozen, they can be wrapped in greaseproof paper and kept in the freezer.

Creamy chocolate lollies

You can coat these in dark chocolate if you are a real chocolate addict (see p212), but these are plain. If you don't want lollies, you can pour the mixture into an ice-cube tray to make mini bites, which are lovely served with a few berries and some cream or yoghurt.

MAKES 6 LOLLIES

NUTRITIONAL INFORMATION PER LOLLY
554 KCALS
51G FAT
8.8G NET CARBOHYDRATES
11.5G PROTEIN

100g dark chocolate (at least 85% cacao content)
250g full-fat Greek yoghurt (I use Total)
250g full-fat cream cheese
250g double cream
50g almond butter (or use any nut butter to suit)
20g almond flakes, crushed
1 tbsp cocoa or cacao powder
2 tbsp erythritol or xylitol (or stevia liquid, to taste)

- Melt the chocolate in a heatproof bowl over a pan of gently simmering water, making sure the base of the bowl doesn't touch the water, or use a microwave for 50 seconds.
- Put the chocolate and the remaining ingredients in a blender or food processor and whizz until smooth.
- Pour into 6 lolly moulds. Freeze until solid (this should take 4–5 hours).

Vanilla ice cream

You need an ice-cream maker for this recipe. This is the base for lots of yummy ice-cream desserts. Add some berries before freezing to turn it into a berry ripple. This recipe uses just egg yolks, but don't throw away the egg whites; pop them into a freezer bag and freeze in batches of two or three, ready to whip up a pavlova or use to make coconut macaroons (page 188). You can also use the egg whites to make an omelette.

MAKES 12 LARGE SCOOPS

NUTRITIONAL INFORMATION PER SCOOP
287 KCALS
29G FAT
2.5G NET CARBOHYDRATES
4G PROTEIN

8 egg yolks
150g erythritol or xylitol
500ml full-fat milk
500ml double or clotted cream
2 vanilla pods

- In a bowl, beat the egg yolks and sweetener together until pale and fluffy.
- Put the milk and cream in a saucepan, and heat over a medium heat. Add the vanilla seeds (cut the pods in half lengthways and use the tip of a knife to scrape out the seeds). I also place the empty pods into the mixture as it all helps to create that lovely vanilla flavour.
- Slowly add a small amount of hot cream to the egg yolks and beat gently – this is the same way we make custard, but do it carefully, a very small amount at a time, as you don't want the eggs to scramble.
- Gradually and very carefully add all the cream and continue to whisk.
- Pour the mixture back into the saucepan and heat over a low heat, stirring all the time until it starts to thicken. Be careful that you don't burn the base.
- Once thickened, remove from the heat and strain into a bowl through a sieve.
- Place a sheet of clingfilm on the custard (so that it touches the custard) as this helps to prevent a skin forming.
- Churn in an ice-cream maker. I have tried to make this without an ice-cream maker, but it becomes hard and icy.

Chocolate ice cream

The secret to this ice cream is the avocados, packed full of goodness and creaminess. Kids love this ice cream and have no idea that it is a healthy option!

SERVES 8

NUTRITIONAL INFORMATION PER SERVING
579 KCALS
59G FAT
4.6G NET CARBOHYDRATES
4.8G PROTEIN

4 ripe avocados, mashed
600ml thick double cream
100g cream cheese
70g erythritol or xylitol (or stevia, to taste)
60g sugar-free cocoa powder or cacao powder

- Put all the ingredients in a food processor and whizz until combined and smooth.
- Pour into a freezer-proof container and freeze for at least 4 hours. If you have an ice-cream maker, you can churn this to make a softer, more whipped ice cream.

Chocolate magic sauce

This is a really simple version of the magic ice-cream sauce that goes hard once it settles onto the ice cream.

SERVES 5

NUTRITIONAL INFORMATION PER 20G SERVING
136 KCALS
12.2G FAT
3.9G NET CARBOHYDRATES
1.5G PROTEIN

100g dark chocolate (at least 85% cacao content)
20g coconut oil

- Put the chocolate and oil in a heatproof bowl over a pan of gently simmering water, making sure the base of the bowl doesn't touch the water, or use a microwave for 50 seconds. Pour over your favourite ice cream.

Savoury Snacks

Here are some savoury nibbles you may enjoy in place of shop-bought crisps and savoury snacks.

Crisps

Although crisps are not laden with sugar, they are refined carbohydrates and not particularly healthy, but sometimes you just want something salty and crispy to crunch on. Pork scratchings, beef jerky and biltong are also good alternatives and readily available in supermarkets.

Parmesan crisps

You can also use Cheddar cheese instead of Parmesan.

MAKES 10 CRISPS

NUTRITIONAL INFORMATION PER CRISP
65 KCALS
4.5G FAT
0G NET CARBOHYDRATES
5.3G PROTEIN

150g Parmesan cheese, grated

- Put 1 tablespoon of grated Parmesan on a sheet of greaseproof paper and spread evenly to form a small circle. There are a couple of ways to cook these crisps: Parmesan works in both the microwave and the oven, but if making Cheddar crisps it is better to bake them in the oven.

Microwave
- Pop into the microwave and cook on full power for 1–2 minutes, depending on the power of your microwave (start at 1 minute and increase by 20-second increments). The Parmesan will melt and bubble – it is done when it has turned slightly golden.
- Remove from the microwave and set aside to cool and set.

Oven
- Bake in the oven at 190°C/gas mark 5 for 10–15 minutes until golden and bubbling. Remove from the oven and set aside to cool and set.

Pepperoni crisps

So simple, but these crisps really hit the spot when you are craving a crunchy, salty, savoury snack. If you want an extra fat/salt hit, you can sprinkle the pepperoni slices with a little Parmesan before baking.

NUTRITIONAL INFORMATION PER 100G
505 KCALS
44G FAT
0G NET CARBOHYDRATES
23G PROTEIN

Pepperoni, finely sliced
Cajun spice blend (page 252)

- Preheat the oven to 190°C/gas mark 5.
- Place the pepperoni slices on a baking tray lined with parchment paper and sprinkle with a little Cajun spice blend.
- Bake for 10 minutes until crispy – timings depend on the thickness of the pepperoni.
- Remove from the oven and, using kitchen paper, dab off the excess fat. Return to the oven for 2 minutes until they crisp up.
- Cool on a wire rack so that they remain crispy – if you leave them on the tray, they may go a bit soft. Store in an airtight container in the fridge.

Crispy bacon crisps

A bit of a basic recipe to be honest, but I do bake these a lot. I have a tub of bacon crisps in the fridge, which is good for an impromptu snack, but they are also great to sprinkle on a salad or to add to egg mayonnaise.

NUTRITIONAL INFORMATION PER 100G
233 KCAL
17G FAT
0G NET CARBOHYDRATES
1.7G PROTEIN

Back bacon rashers

- Preheat the oven to 180°C/gas mark 4.
- Put the bacon rashers on a baking tray lined with parchment paper and bake for 10–15 minutes until really crispy – timings depend on the thickness of the bacon.
- Allow to cool, then cut into pieces. Store in an airtight container in the fridge for 3 to 4 days.

Kale crisps

These are really tasty, so do try them. You can coat them with whichever spice you like, ranging from chilli, garlic or even nutritional yeast flakes, which impart a cheesy flavour. You can keep things quite simple and opt for sea salt, black pepper and paprika as this gives a simple flavour that is also suitable for children, but the combination below is my personal favourite.

Note: I was sent a dehydrator from Lakeland to review, which I seriously recommend. It saves popping them in the oven and the crisps come out drier and crisper.

NUTRITIONAL INFORMATION PER 100G
107 KCALS
7.2G FAT
0.81G NET CARBOHYDRATES
1.4G PROTEIN

200g kale
1 tbsp olive oil or melted coconut oil
Sea salt
Freshly ground black pepper
1 tsp paprika
1 tsp garlic powder
½ tsp dried thyme
½ tsp chilli powder

- Preheat the oven to 150°C/gas mark 2. Line a baking tray with baking parchment.
- Wash and dry the kale, making sure it is perfectly dry. Remove the stems and thick bits, leaving the nice leaves.
- Put the kale in a bowl with the oil and flavourings. Mix well to ensure it is all evenly coated.
- Spread the kale on the baking tray and bake for 20–30 minutes. Turn off the oven and leave the kale in the oven to dry out more. Allow to cool, then store in an airtight container for 2 to 4 days.

Parmesan tacos

The method shown here is for the microwave, but you can make these in the oven – just be careful that they don't burn! Cook for 5–8 minutes at 170°C until golden and bubbling. Serve with Low-carb Chili (see p104)

MAKES 4 TACOS

NUTRITIONAL INFO PER TACO
262 KCALS
19G FAT
0.6G NET CARBOHYDRATES
22G PROTEIN

250g Parmesan cheese, grated

- Place 2–4 tablespoons of Parmesan on a sheet of greaseproof paper and spread evenly to form a circle.
- Pop into the microwave and cook on full power for 1–2 minutes, depending on the power of your microwave (start at 1 minute and increase by 20 seconds). The Parmesan will melt and bubble – the taco is done when it has gone slightly golden.
- Remove from the microwave, but keep on the greaseproof paper and immediately place over the side of a bottle or rolling pin, pulling the sides down to create a taco shape. Leave until cool and it will set into shape. Alternatively, place into a bowl to form your own Parmesan bowl shape.

Finger-licking almonds

These are really moreish, so you have been warned! I like to make them when I get a craving for crisps – usually, if I am honest, when I am enjoying a little tipple!

NUTRITIONAL INFORMATION PER 100G
621 KCALS
54G FAT
6.7G NET CARBOHYDRATES
15G FIBRE
18.7G PROTEIN

300g whole blanched almonds
1–2 tsp chilli powder, to taste
1 tsp garlic powder
1 tsp dried thyme
2 tsp paprika
Generous sprinkle of sea salt
Freshly ground black pepper
1 tbsp olive oil or melted coconut oil

- Preheat the oven to 170°C/gas mark 3.
- Put all in the ingredients in a bowl and combine, ensuring the almonds are evenly coated. Tip onto a baking tray and bake for 8 minutes. Allow to cool, then store in an airtight container for up to a couple of weeks.

Sweet cinnamon nuts

These are really nice to have on top of natural yoghurt. They are also nice with chopped apple. They remind me of the flavours of Christmas.

NUTRITIONAL INFORMATION PER 100G
637 KCALS
55G FAT
6.7G NET CARBOHYDRATES
18.9G PROTEIN

300g mixed nuts (almonds, pecans, walnuts and Macadamia nuts)
2 tbsp coconut oil, melted
2 tsp ground cinnamon, plus extra if needed
1 tsp allspice
1 tsp mixed spice
2 tsp Sukrin Gold (optional)

- Preheat the oven to 150°C/gas mark 2.
- Put the nuts in a bowl and mix in the coconut oil, spices and Sukrin Gold, if using.
- Tip onto a baking tray and spread out so that they are in a single layer.
- You can finish with a sprinkling of cinnamon if you are unsure whether they are evenly coated. Bake for 5–8 minutes – no more or they will start to burn.
- Allow to cool, then store in an airtight container for up to a couple of weeks.

Confectionary and Sweet Treats

This chapter demonstrates that you can have your sweets and treats when you are on a sugar-free lifestyle, but it is also important to emphasise that I don't want you to binge on these! As your palate changes, you will be less and less reliant on the sweet treats. There is a risk if you have too many sweet foods that you may start craving sugary snacks, and I really don't want to encourage that.

Chocolate facts

You will need to opt for dark chocolate for all these recipes, ideally with as much cacao content as you can find. Check the sugar content, as it does vary between brands. You can also buy sugar-free chocolate sweetened with stevia or xylitol.

I melt chocolate in a microwave, using the Lakeland silicon melting pot, but you can use a bain-marie method if you prefer. The typical way of doing this, though, is to melt the chocolate in a heatproof bowl over a pan of gently simmering water, making sure the base of the bowl doesn't touch the water. I microwave the chocolate in 30 second intervals, making sure it does not burn.

I love using silicon chocolate moulds. You can pick these up really cheaply and they give your chocolates a professional look. I use a paintbrush to help coat the moulds, refrigerating or freezing them between each coating.

Sweetness does vary depending on personal taste, so my suggestions are guidelines only. As you get used to a sugar-free lifestyle, you will find you rely less and less on natural sweeteners.

As mentioned in the opening chapters, stevia can leave a lingering aftertaste. I use liquid stevia, but the aftertaste does vary depending on the brand and your own personal susceptibility. You can opt for flavoured stevia liquid, which can be quite helpful for recipes in this chapter. If in doubt, opt for xylitol or erythritol blend.

Remember, opt for strong dark chocolate and use less sugar – your palate will soon get used to this. Try not to be too reliant on adding these treats to your diet – they are treats and not everyday foods.

Chocolate mint creams

You can make these on a baking tray and cut them into squares before dipping them into chocolate, or if you want to be a bit fancy, why not use a silicon chocolate mould (which I prefer). Coat the moulds with dark chocolate before adding the filling, then cover again with chocolate (see p228). Freeze between each stage to speed up the process.

MAKES 20 MINT CREAMS

NUTRITIONAL INFORMATION PER CHOCOLATE
117 KCALS
11.2G FAT
2.5G NET CARBOHYDRATES
1G PROTEIN

200g dark chocolate (at least 85% cacao content)
100g coconut oil, melted
75g extra-thick cream
1 tsp peppermint extract
2–5 drops of liquid stevia, to taste, or 2–3 tsp erythritol or xylitol (optional)

- Melt the chocolate in a heatproof bowl over a pan of gently simmering water, making sure the base of the bowl doesn't touch the water, or use a microwave (this takes seconds).
- Line a 20cm square brownie tin with greaseproof paper. Pour half the chocolate into the tin and spread evenly. Place in the fridge or freezer until set. Alternatively, you can line silicon chocolate moulds with the chocolate and place in the fridge or the freezer until set.
- Mix the melted coconut oil with the cream and peppermint extract. The mixture will curdle at first, but keep stirring with a small hand whisk or fork. It will start to thicken as it cools. Add the sweetener if you prefer a sweeter taste.
- Pour the mint mixture onto the set chocolate base (or fill the chocolate moulds) and return to the fridge or freezer to set.
- Cover with the remaining chocolate and refrigerate/freeze until set.
- If using a brownie tin, remove from the tin and cut into small squares. Place in an airtight container in the fridge for up to 5 days.

Sugar-free faux Ferrero Rocher

I must confess that I had very little to do with this recipe. My son decided to make my sugar-free chocolate spread. I left him to it and only intervened when he shouted that the mixture was too thick. He had blended everything together instead of blending the hazelnuts first, so we ended up with a thick, chocolate mixture with a combination of whole and blended hazelnuts. It tasted amazing and we soon realised it was exactly like Ferrero Rocher! We made these into balls and coated them with chocolate. How wonderful!

I don't use sweetener in this recipe, but feel free to add a small amount of stevia liquid if you feel it needs it.

MAKES 20 CHOCOLATES

NUTRITIONAL INFORMATION PER CHOCOLATE
146 KCALS
13.5G FAT
2.5G NET CARBOHYDRATES
2.5G PROTEIN

For the balls
200g blanched hazelnuts (plus 20 hazelnuts for centres)
75g dark chocolate (at least 85% cacao content)
30g coconut oil
1 tbsp unsweetened cocoa or cacao powder
1 tsp sugar-free vanilla extract (optional)
2–5 drops of stevia liquid, to taste (optional)

To coat
75g dark chocolate (at least 85% cacao content)
30g coconut oil
20g blanched hazelnuts, finely chopped

- Preheat the oven to 160°C/gas mark 2½.
- Start by making the balls. Put the hazelnuts for the balls and the centres on a baking tray and roast for 8–10 minutes. When the nuts are warm they release their oils better, making a much smoother spread.
- Meanwhile, melt the chocolate and coconut oil in a heatproof bowl over a pan of gently simmering water, making sure the base of the bowl doesn't touch the water, or use a microwave for 50 seconds.
- Put all the ingredients for the balls in a blender or food processor and blend until smooth. Put the nuts for the centres to one side.
- Scrape out into a bowl. Form the mixture into balls, then pop a hazelnut into each ball. Place on a sheet of greaseproof paper. Refrigerate for 20 minutes.
- To make the coating, melt the chocolate and coconut oil together. Dip the balls into the chocolate (I place each ball on the end of a fork and dip it into the chocolate) or pour the chocolate over the balls – whatever you find easier. Sprinkle with chopped hazelnuts and refrigerate until set.

Top tip: For ease of use, I used blanched hazelnuts, but if you use ones with the skin on you will have to remove these before blending. Do this after they come out of the oven: put them in a freezer bag and shake/roll them to remove most of the skins.

Chocolate orange creams

I make these in silicon chocolate moulds as they look really lovely. The orange flavour depends on the type of flavouring used. I have tried several and they do vary, so the key is to taste as you go – too much flavouring can give an artificial taste. For adults only, why not add some Cointreau to the mixture?

MAKES 20 ORANGE CREAMS

NUTRITIONAL INFORMATION PER CHOCOLATE
117 KCALS
11.2G FAT
2.5G NET CARBOHYDRATES
1G PROTEIN

200g dark chocolate (at least 85% cacao content)
100g coconut oil
60g thick double cream
Orange flavouring, to taste
2–5 drops of stevia liquid or sweetener of choice (optional)
Orange food colouring (optional)

- Melt the chocolate in a microwave or in a heatproof bowl over simmering water.
- Coat the silicon moulds with chocolate. I use a brush to do this.
- Place in the fridge or freezer to set. You may wish to line the moulds again with another layer of chocolate. If so, refrigerate again to set.
- Melt the coconut oil and stir in the cream. The mixture will curdle at first, but use a fork or whisk and it will come together. As it cools it will thicken up a lot more.
- Add the orange flavouring, sweetener (if using) and optional colouring. If you are using Cointreau, add 1–2 tablespoons, to taste, to the mixture now. Taste as you go to achieve the strength of flavour and sweetness that suits you.
- Remove the moulds from the fridge and fill with the mixture. Refrigerate for a further 10 minutes to set.
- Add the final chocolate coating before placing them back into the fridge.
- Once set, turn out and pop into an airtight container and keep in the fridge for up to 5 days.

Dark chocolate coconut bars

These coconut bars are really easy to make and kids love them. They also store well in the freezer so you can make a big batch of them at once.

MAKES 8 BARS

NUTRITIONAL INFORMATION PER BAR
362 KCALS
33.6G FAT
7.1G NET CARBOHYDRATES
4G PROTEIN

200g desiccated coconut
30g coconut oil, melted
1–2 tbsp Surkin fibre syrup or rice malt syrup (or stevia, to taste)
60g coconut cream
175g dark chocolate (at least 85% cacao content) (or raw cacao)

- Combine all the ingredients, apart from the chocolate, in a bowl.
- Mould into eight small bars and place on a baking tray. Place the tray in the freezer until the mixture is frozen.
- Melt the chocolate in a heatproof bowl over a pan of gently simmering water, making sure the base of the bowl doesn't touch the water, or use a microwave (this takes seconds).
- Remove the coconut bars from the freezer and coat them with the chocolate: you can dip these into the chocolate or coat one side at a time, turning once set.
- Place on a sheet of baking parchment and refrigerate or freeze until set. Store in an airtight container in the fridge for up to 5 days or freezer.

Chocolate pecan bark

You can sprinkle the chocolate with a variety of nuts, seeds or fruit, so feel free to adapt to suit your taste or what is in your store cupboard.

MAKES ABOUT 12 SQUARES

NUTRITIONAL INFORMATION PER SQUARE
125 KCALS
10.9G FAT
4G NET CARBOHYDRATES
1.7G PROTEIN

200g dark chocolate (at least 80% cacao content)
2 tsp coconut oil
20g pecan nuts, roughly crushed
Sprinkle of sea salt (optional)

- Line a 25cm square tin with baking parchment.
- Melt the chocolate and coconut oil together in a heatproof bowl over a pan of gently simmering water, making sure the base of the bowl doesn't touch the water, or use a microwave (this takes seconds).
- Pour into the prepared tin, spreading evenly with a palate knife.
- Sprinkle on the nuts, pushing them down slightly to secure them into the chocolate. Sprinkle over a little sea salt, if using.
- Refrigerate for at least 1 hour, then cut into 12 squares. Store in an airtight container in the fridge.

Coconut ice

I used to eat this as a child, but I think my mum used condensed milk in her recipe. It was probably packed with sugar! This recipe is sugar free but is well worth a try and is so easy to make.

MAKES 30 SQUARES

NUTRITIONAL INFORMATION PER SQUARE
200 KCALS
20G FAT
1.6G NET CARBOHYDRATES
1.5G PROTEIN

400g coconut milk
150g coconut oil
100g erythritol or xylitol
600g desiccated coconut

- Line a 22cm square brownie tin with baking parchment.
- Put the milk and coconut oil in a saucepan and heat until melted and combined.
- Add the sweetener and stir until dissolved.
- Remove from the heat and stir in the desiccated coconut, ensuring it is evenly coated in the milky mixture.
- Transfer the mixture to the prepared tin. Refrigerate for at least 3 hours to set, then slice into 30 squares.

Top tip: You can colour half the mixture to create the traditional pink and white coconut ice.

Chocolate fudge

This is easy to prepare and is a nice treat, especially at Christmas. I have bagged these and given them away as gifts for friends and clients who are low carb.

MAKES 12 SQUARES

NUTRITIONAL INFORMATION PER SQUARE
314 KCALS
31G FAT
2.8G NET CARBOHYDRATES
4.2G PROTEIN

175g coconut oil
75g dark chocolate (at least 90% cacao content)
200g almond butter
100g double cream
1 tbsp sugar-free cocoa powder
1 tsp sugar-free vanilla extract (optional)

- Line a 12cm square Pyrex dish with baking parchment.
- Melt the coconut oil and chocolate in a heatproof bowl over a pan of gently simmering water, making sure the base of the bowl doesn't touch the water, or use a microwave (this takes seconds). Add to a blender with the remaining ingredients and whizz until smooth.
- Pour into the prepared dish and even out, then refrigerate for at least 3 hours to set.
- Cut into 12 squares and store in an airtight container in the fridge.

Gelatine jellied sweets

Gelatine doesn't sound very attractive, does it? And it doesn't sound like an ingredient whose use is to be encouraged, but think again. Gelatine helps promote the right environment for healthy bacteria in the gut. It is also very protective of the digestive tract. It can improve joint health and strengthen hair and nails. I use grass-fed beef gelatine powder, but the choice is yours. If you use gelatine sheets, place them in cold water to go limp before adding them to the warm liquid.

Top tip: You can buy fantastic silicon moulds online (Amazon and Lakeland are my favourites) in all shapes and sizes. I love the jelly-baby moulds. I also fill these with left-over smoothies and freeze them. They are great to serve with some berries, and kids love them!

Sugar-free berry jelly bears

If you are using raspberries or strawberries, you may want to sieve them before adding them to the liquid to remove the pips.

MAKES 24

NUTRITIONAL INFORMATION PER JELLY BEAR
11.2 KCALS
0.01G FAT
0.16G NET CARBOHYDRATES
2.4G PROTEIN

80g fresh or frozen berries of your choice
200ml water (or full-fat milk or coconut water)
30g erythritol or xylitol (or a few drops of stevia liquid, to taste)
Juice of ½ lemon
3 tbsp gelatine

- I use my NutriBullet to pulp the fruit (adding a little water to help blend) but you can use a blender or just mush together as thoroughly as you can until you have a smooth pulp.
- In a saucepan over a medium heat, heat the water, sweetener and lemon juice until warm. Add the gelatine and stir with a whisk until combined and the water starts to look a bit glossy and smooth.
- Add the fruit purée and combine well, then pour into silicon moulds. This is not as easy as it sounds, so ensure that you use a jug with a nice pouring action or it could get messy! I place my moulds onto a baking sheet before adding the liquid to keep them stable for when I transport them to the fridge.
- Leave in the fridge until set.

The Pantry

Stocks and gravy

Bone broth/stock

This is a really healthy broth – much better for you than processed stock cubes. It is packed with minerals such as calcium, magnesium and phosphorus. It helps to support the digestive tract, boosts the immune system and reduces inflammation, as well as strengthening joints, hair and nails and promoting healthy skin. Speak to your butcher as they are often happy to give away bones for you to use.

Invest in a large stock pot so that you can make up several litres at a time and store it in the fridge or freezer. I store stock in freezer bags as well as large silicon ice moulds. The freezer bags can be defrosted quickly by popping the sealed bag into a bowl of water. I use the silicon moulds to pop out a few small 'ice stocks' to add to dishes such as a chilli or spaghetti bolognaise.

Use a large stock pot (or you could use a slow cooker or even a pressure cooker).

1kg bones (bone marrow, ribs, knuckles, etc.)
200ml apple cider vinegar
2 large onions, chopped into quarters
2 cloves of garlic, cut into chunks
2 carrots, cut into chunks (optional)
2 sticks of celery, cut into chunks
2 tsp dried mixed herbs
Small handful of parsley (or 2–3 tsp dried)
2 bay leaves
2 tsp peppercorns

- If using meaty bones, roast them in the oven at 190°C/gas mark 5 for 45 minutes to help release the flavours and nutrients. You can omit this step if you prefer.
- Put all the ingredients into a stock pot and cover with cold water. Simmer for 24–48 hours for beef bones, or 12–24 hours for chicken bones.
- You may want to remove any scum from the surface of the water occasionally. I use a slotted spoon to scoop it out.
- Remove from the heat and strain. A layer of fat will form on the top once cooled and settled. Don't discard this; use it as a cooking fat.
- Transfer to a jar, freezer bag or silicon ice moulds ready to use in everyday savoury dishes.

Spreads, jams and chutneys

Hazelnutty chocolate spread

It is disgusting the amount of sugar, palm oil and skimmed milk powder found in commercial chocolate spreads, yet they still claim they are good for you! This is a really easy recipe that will satisfy the chocolate addict in everyone. It is sugar free and sweetener free as I really don't think it needs anything else; however, if you have a very sweet tooth, you can add some rice malt syrup or a drop or two of stevia liquid to taste – although beware, you need to start adjusting your palate to less sweet options, and this is a fantastic start!

At the time of writing, the leading brand in chocolate spread contains a huge 56.8g of sugar per 100g – that's almost 60% sugar!

MAKES 1 JAR (ABOUT 500G)

NUTRITIONAL INFORMATION PER 1 TBSP SERVING
102 KCALS
9.6 FAT
1.4G NET CARBOHYDRATES (0.8 SUGAR)
1.8G PROTEIN

350g blanched hazelnuts
100g dark chocolate (at least 85% cacao content), melted
2 tbsp coconut oil, melted
1 tsp sugar-free vanilla extract
1–2 tbsp erythritol or xylitol (or stevia drops, to taste) (optional)

- Preheat the oven to 160°C/gas mark 3.
- Put the hazelnuts on a baking tray and roast for 8–10 minutes. When nuts are warm they release their oils better, making a much smoother spread.
- Put the hazelnuts in a blender or food processor and blend until smooth.
- Melt the chocolate and coconut oil together in the microwave, in 20-second bursts until melted, then add this to the blender along with the vanilla. Blend until smooth.
- If you want a sweeter chocolate, add a few erythritol, xylitol or stevia drops. If you add sweetener it will thicken the chocolate spread.
- Store in sterilised jars. It will go hard when refrigerated, so the spread is best served at room temperature.

Raspberry chia jam

My mum makes a wonderful raspberry jam, using less than half the sugar of conventional jams, which I love. The sharpness of flavour is fantastic. I don't add any sweetener to this as I don't think it needs it, but feel free to add xylitol, erythritol or stevia, to taste. This takes minutes to make and will keep for 2–3 weeks if refrigerated and stored in a sterilised jar. You can also use strawberries or blueberries.

MAKES 1 SMALL JAR (ABOUT 200G)

NUTRITIONAL INFORMATION PER 1 TBSP SERVING
18.5 KCALS
0.9G FAT
0.8G NET CARBOHYDRATES
0.7G PROTEIN

200g raspberries (frozen work brilliantly)
2 tbsp chia seeds

- Put the raspberries in a saucepan and heat over a medium heat, slightly squishing them as they warm.
- When the raspberries start to break down and release their juices, add the chia seeds. Stir for 1–2 minutes – the jam will start to thicken as the chia absorb the liquid.
- Pour into a sterilised jar and store in the fridge for up to 3 weeks.

Lemon curd

I make this in the slow cooker as I find it so easy. If you don't want to make it in a slow cooker, you can do it in a bain-marie, dramatically reducing the cooking time.

MAKES 2 JARS (ABOUT 500G)

NUTRITIONAL INFORMATION PER 1 TBSP SERVING
196 KCALS
21G FAT
0.8G NET CARBOHYDRATES
0.4G PROTEIN

100g butter
100g erythritol or xylitol (add more if you prefer it sweeter)
Zest and juice of 4 large lemons, pips removed
4 eggs

- Place the butter, sweetener, lemon zest and juice in a 1.2-litre pudding basin. Place in the slow cooker on low. Pour boiling water around the bowl until it comes halfway up the side.
- Leave for 20 minutes. Remove from the slow cooker and leave to cool for 5 minutes. Keep the slow cooker on, as you will be returning the basin shortly.
- Beat the eggs and pour through a sieve over the bowl of lemon mixture, beating all the time.
- Secure a piece of foil over the basin and seal well with string.
- Return the basin to the slow cooker, keeping the temperature low. Add more boiling water around the basin, ensuring the water comes more than halfway up the side of the bowl.
- Cook for 2–3 hours, stirring a couple of times to avoid lumps (if you forget to stir and the mixture goes lumpy or curdles, whisk it well with a balloon whisk after cooking).
- The curd should be thick enough to coat the back of a spoon, but not thick and lumpy. Pour into sterilised jars. Cover with a layer of parchment before sealing with the lid.
- Keep refrigerated once opened.

Blueberry jam

A lovely jam, this is perfect spread on slices of Lemon Drizzle Cake (page 181). It takes minutes to make and will keep for 2–3 weeks if refrigerated and stored in a sterilised jar.

MAKES 1 SMALL JAR (ABOUT 200G)

NUTRITIONAL INFORMATION PER 1 TBSP SERVING
12.8 KCALS
0.53G FAT
1.1G NET CARBOHYDRATES
0.4G PROTEIN

200g fresh blueberries
Zest and juice of 1 lemon
1–2 tsp erythritol or xylitol (or stevia, to taste) (optional)
2 tbsp chia seeds

- Put the blueberries in a saucepan and heat over a medium heat, slightly squishing the blueberries as they warm. Add the lemon zest, juice and 50ml cold water.
- Cook for 10 minutes over a low heat until the blueberries release their juices and start to break down. If you prefer a sweeter jam, add the sweetener.
- Stir in the chia seeds for 2–4 minutes. The jam will start to thicken as the chia seeds absorb the liquid. Pour into a sterilised jar and store in the fridge for up to 3 weeks.

Fresh tomato relish

This relish can only be made fresh and will last no more than 2–3 days in the fridge. It makes a really nice topping for meat, fish or even burgers, and it adds a nice flavour to a salad, especially when topped with feta cheese.

MAKES 2 JARS (ABOUT 1KG)

NUTRITIONAL INFORMATION PER 1 TBSP SERVING
13 KCALS
1.1G FAT
0.5G NET CARBOHYDRATES
0.1G PROTEIN

750g tomatoes, diced
6 sun-dried tomatoes, diced
6 spring onions, finely chopped
½ red pepper, deseeded and finely diced
2 cloves of garlic, crushed
1 chilli, finely chopped
Small handful of fresh parsley
Small handful of fresh chives
6 tbsp extra-virgin olive oil
3 tbsp white wine vinegar
Freshly ground black pepper

- Place all the vegetables and herbs in a bowl and combine.
- Mix the oil and vinegar together and season with black pepper. Pour this over the vegetables and herbs, combine well and store in the fridge for up to 3 days.

Tomato ketchup

This ketchup does take a while to cook as it needs to reduce, but it is worth it. It will keep stored in airtight sterilised jars for up to 6 months. I store mine in the fridge.

MAKES ABOUT 1KG

NUTRITIONAL INFORMATION PER 1 TBSP SERVING
7.3 KCALS
0.3G FAT
0.7G NET CARBOHYDRATES
0.2G PROTEIN

1 tsp coconut oil or 1 tbsp olive oil
1 large red onion, peeled and diced
1 stick of celery, diced
½ carrot, diced
2 cloves of garlic, sliced
½ red chilli, deseeded and finely chopped (optional)
500g cherry tomatoes, diced
400g tin chopped tomatoes
8 sun-dried tomatoes
3 tsp tomato purée
1 tsp paprika
½ tsp onion powder
½ tsp garlic powder
½ tsp dried oregano
1 bay leaf
150ml apple cider vinegar
300ml water
70g Sukrin Gold, or to taste
Salt and freshly ground black pepper

- Put the coconut oil in a heavy-based saucepan and heat over a medium heat. Add the onion, celery, carrot, garlic and chilli.
- Cook gently for 5 minutes to soften, then add the tomatoes.
- Cook for a further 5–10 minutes, or until the tomatoes start to break down and ooze their juices. Add all the remaining ingredients and season to taste.
- Cook gently until the mixture has reduced by about half. This may take up to 45 minutes. Don't be tempted to increase the temperature above a medium heat, as you don't want the mixture to burn.
- Remove the bay leaf. Use a stick blender and whizz until smooth – you can use a liquidiser if you prefer. If you like a fine sauce, pop it through a sieve before returning it to the saucepan.
- If the sauce is not thick enough, either give it a longer cook or you can add some cornflour (mix 1 tablespoon with a little water to form a paste before stirring it into the mixture). Low carb/grain free can use coconut flour or xanthan gum.
- When it is at the right thickness, taste and season again if needed. If you find it too acidic, add a little more sweetener or a few more sun-dried tomatoes. Store in sterilised jars.

Note: You can make this in the slow cooker, but you'll need to sauté the vegetables before putting them in the slow cooker and omit the water. Cook on low for 6–8 hours.

Easy mayonnaise

You can make this with a stick blender or a food processor. I make a basic mayonnaise, then add seasoning and other flavourings, such as garlic or chilli, after I've made the base. This gives me the flexibility to make up several flavours to store in small containers.

MAKES 1 JAR (ABOUT 400G)

NUTRITIONAL INFORMATION PER 1 TBSP SERVING
16.5 KCALS
12.8G FAT
0G NET CARBOHYDRATES
0G PROTEIN

2 egg yolks
300ml olive oil
Salt and freshly ground black pepper

- Put the egg yolks in a tall container and whisk with a stick blender, then add the oil, drizzle by drizzle. Continue whisking until you have the consistency you require. Season to taste.

Sun-dried tomato and basil pesto

If you love pesto but don't want the added cheese, this recipe is perfect. It delivers great flavour, perfect as a topping for a healthy pizza or stuffed in a chicken breast.

MAKES 1 SMALL JAR (ABOUT 6 SERVINGS)

NUTRITIONAL INFORMATION PER 1 TBSP SERVING
138 KCALS
14G FAT
1G NET CARBOHYDRATES
1.4G PROTEIN

125g sun-dried tomatoes
Large handful of fresh basil
75g pine nuts
3–4 cloves of garlic, to taste
4 tbsp extra-virgin olive oil
Salt and freshly ground black pepper

- Put all the ingredients in a food processor or blender and whizz until smooth.
- Pour into a bowl, cover and refrigerate for at least 30 minutes, allowing the flavours to infuse.
- Store in an airtight container in the fridge for up to 1 week. You can also freeze this. I usually pour it into a silicon ice-cube tray and pop out a few cubes when I need them.

Sun-dried tomato paste

Just like spices, sadly, shop-bought sun-dried tomato paste contains unwanted sugar. This is really simple to make yourself. You can store it in a jar or even place it in a silicon ice mould, ready to pop out 'sun-dried tomato' bales whenever you need to add some to a dish.

Note: I ask you to drain the sun-dried tomatoes from the oil in the jar because it is often vegetable or sunflower oil and it is far healthier to have olive oil in your food.

MAKES 1 SMALL JAR (ABOUT 150G)

NUTRITIONAL INFORMATION PER 1 TBSP SERVING
47 KCALS
3.2G FAT
3.1G NET CARBOHYDRATES
0.7G PROTEIN

Jar of sun-dried tomatoes, drained, leaving about 150g
2 cloves of garlic
1 tsp dried oregano
3 tbsp olive oil
Salt and freshly ground pepper

- Whizz all the ingredients in a food processor until smooth. Store in a sterilised jar in the fridge for up to 1 week or freeze in silicon ice moulds.

Red Thai paste

This is a nice paste that can add flavour to a lot of dishes. Add it to chicken, soups or noodles. If you are serving this to children, you may want to adjust the chilli content.

MAKES 1 SMALL JAR (ABOUT 100G)

NUTRITIONAL INFORMATION PER 1 TBSP SERVING
31 KCALS
2.7G FAT
0.9G NET CARBOHYDRATES
0.4G PROTEIN

4 tbsp olive oil
3 red or green chillies, finely chopped
4 cloves of garlic
½ red onion
1 piece of fresh ginger, peeled
3 stalks of lemongrass
Juice and zest of 1 lime
3 tbsp paprika
3 tsp cumin seeds
3 tsp coriander seeds
3 sun-dried tomatoes
Small bunch of fresh coriander

- Put all the ingredients in a food processor and whizz to a paste.
- Store in a sterilised jar and refrigerate for up to 2–3 weeks.

Spice blends

It is a sad fact that most of the spice blends in our supermarkets contain added sugar. It is frustrating as we really don't need it and it's time food manufacturers recognised this. However, in the meantime, do as I do and make up your own spice blends and store them in small airtight jars until needed. The quantities can be doubled or even tripled if you want to store them in larger jars.

Southern chicken spice mix

150g ground almonds or ground pork scratchings
4 tsp paprika
2 tsp dried parsley
3 tsp chicken bouillon or 4 tsp chicken seasoning (ensure sugar free)
2 tsp dried oregano
1 tsp dried tarragon
2 tsp dried thyme
2 tsp garlic powder
1 tsp onion salt
1 tsp celery salt
Salt and freshly ground black pepper

Fajita seasoning

4 tsp chilli powder
4 tsp garlic powder
6 tsp paprika
4 tsp dried oregano
2 tsp ground cumin
4 tsp onion powder
2 tsp dried parsley

Cajun spice mix

2 tsp garlic powder
3 tsp paprika
1 tsp onion powder
1 tsp cayenne pepper
2 tsp dried oregano
1 tsp chilli powder
½ tsp salt
½ tsp freshly ground black pepper

Curry powder

6 tsp ground coriander
3 tsp cumin
4 tsp turmeric
1 tsp ground mustard seeds
½ tsp ground ginger
1 tsp chilli powder (add more if you like it very hot)
½ tsp garlic powder
½ tsp onion powder
½ tsp grated nutmeg
½ tsp cayenne pepper

Moroccan seasoning

3 tsp paprika
1 tsp ground cinnamon
½ tsp garlic powder
½ tsp onion powder
1 tsp ground cumin
2 tsp ground coriander
½ tsp cayenne pepper
½ tsp allspice

Italian seasoning

4 tsp dried oregano
2 tsp dried thyme
1 tsp dried basil
4 tsp dried parsley
1 tsp garlic powder
½ tsp onion powder

References

This is a list of my favourite resources for sugar-free and LCHF (also known as banting and keto). YouTube is an excellent starting point to watch videos of these experts, but do also take the time to look at their websites and subscribe to their newsletters and Facebook pages. I have also listed some books that I would highly recommend.

Remember, education and knowledge are keys to success.

> 'Knowledge is power. Information is liberating. Education is the premise of progress, in every society, in every family.'
> **Kofi Annan, former Secretary-General of the United Nations**

Key figures in the LCHF/banting/keto world

Professor Tim Noakes

A South African scientist, Tim Noakes is one of the best pioneers for the low-carb movement. You can find him on Twitter @ProfTimNoakes and find out more about his work with The Noakes Foundation at www.thenoakesfoundation.org. I would also highly recommend his latest book, *Lore of Nutrition: Challenging Conventional Dietary Beliefs.*

The Diet Doctor

Dr Andreas Eenfeldt is a Swedish medical doctor whose aim is to spread the word about our outdated nutritional information and push for a food revolution. I cannot recommend his book *Low Carb, High Fat Food Revolution* highly enough. It is a very easy read and details why we are facing the health epidemics we are seeing today. He has some fantastic lectures on YouTube, and I would highly recommend subscribing to his website for meal plans and access to some excellent films, advice and case studies. www.dietdoctor.com

Dr Jason Fung

A fantastic doctor, Jason Fung makes every lecture fun and easy to understand. He is passionate about combining the benefits of fasting with a low-carb diet to ensure solid results, especially with those suffering from Type 2 diabetes and obesity. I highly recommend watching his lectures on YouTube. You can also buy his excellent book on obesity, *The Obesity Code*, and his must-read book on fasting, *The Complete Guide to Fasting.*

Dr Zoe Harcombe

Zoe Harcombe is a speaker, author, researcher and campaigner for real food. Her website is fantastic, tackling some hard-hitting topics incredibly thoroughly. Zoe was also involved in the creation of the brilliant book *Diabetes Unpacked*. www.zoeharcombe.com

Dr Eric Berg

Eric Berg is an American doctor who offers some really fascinating videos on health and keto. Worth a look. www.drberg.com

Dr Robert Lustig

Another fascinating American doctor, Robert Lustig specialises in paediatric endocrinology. He has published some fantastic books, including *Fat Chance: The Hidden Truth about Sugar* and *The Hacking of the American Mind*. It is also worth watching the film *Fed-up*, an American documentary, which features Dr Robert Lustig.

Gary Taubes

If you are interested in the science and research behind sugar, Gary is your man. He has some fascinating lectures on YouTube and several great books such as *Why We Get Fat*, *Good Calories, Bad Calories* and *The Case Against Sugar*.

Dr Gary Fettke

Gary and his wife Belinda Fettke are based in Australia. Gary is an orthopaedic surgeon and is passionate about the low-carb way of eating to help reverse Type 2 diabetes. Visit their website: www.nofructose.com.

Dr Aseem Malhotra

A really inspiring cardiologist, Aseem Malhotra is passionate about promoting real food, sugar-free and a low-carb Mediterranean lifestyle. His book, *The Pioppi Diet*, is a bestseller. He regularly appears in the media and his lectures are well worth watching. Also check out the three films: *Cereal Killers 1*, *Cereal Killers 2: Run on Fat* and *Big Fat Fix*, which features Dr Malhotra.

Public Health Collaboration

This is a fantastic charity dedicated to informing and implementing healthy decisions for better public health alongside the promotion of real food. I would highly recommend joining and attending their fascinating conferences. www.phcuk.org.

Diabetes.co.uk

This website offers a fantastic, free low-carb programme, which has been put together by the amazing GP, Dr David Unwin, featured in the opening chapters of this book.

Other great books include *The Big Fat Surprise* by Nina Teicholz and *The Great Cholesterol Con* by Malcolm Kendrick.

Index